PREVENTION'S

Medical Care Yearbook

1989

By the Editors of *Prevention*® Magazine

Edited by Sharon Stocker Ferguson

Senior Research Associate, *Prevention*® Magazine

Rodale Press, Emmaus, Pennsylvania

Chapter 16, "Is Calcium a Cancer Preventer?" was adapted from *The Calcium Connection: A Revolutionary Diet and Health Program to Reduce Hypertension, Prevent Osteoporosis, and Lower the Risk of Cancer,* by Cedric Garland, Ph.D, and Frank Garland, Ph.D., with Ellen Thro and with the assistance of Eve Garliano (New York: G. P. Putnam's Sons, 1988). Reprinted by permission of the publisher.

Chapter 19, "How to Tell Your Doctor What Hurts," was adapted from *Get Well, Stay Well: The Successful Patient's Handbook,* by Barry Gordon, M.D. (New York: Dembner Books, 1988). Reprinted by permission of the publisher.

Chapter 20, "Shoot Down the Flu," was adapted from *Cold Cures: The Medical Self-Care Guide to Prevention and Treatment of the Common Cold and Flu,* by Michael Castleman (New York: Ballantine Books, 1987). Reprinted by permission of the author.

Chapter 25, "The D and C: Make Sure You Need It," was adapted from *Women under the Knife,* by Herbert H. Keyser, M.D. (Philadelphia: George F. Stickley, 1984). Reprinted by permission of the author.

Chapter 38, "When Food Becomes a Foe," was adapted from "A Parent's Guide to Childhood Allergies," by Paula Brisco, originally published in *Children* magazine (June 1988). Reprinted by permission of the author.

Chapter 39, "Modern Management of Childhood Asthma," was adapted from "Happy and Healthy Despite Asthma," by Mary Blakinger, originally published in *Children* magazine (Winter 1987). Reprinted by permission of the author.

The following chapters were adapted from and reprinted by permission of *Medical Self-Care* magazine, P.O. Box 1000, Pt. Reyes, CA 94956 (free sample magazine available on request): Chapter 2, "Alternative 'Medicine' for Back Pain" ("The New Back Care," July–August 1987); Chapter 26, "Battling Lupus" ("Lupus," March–April 1988); and Chapter 27, "Vaginitis Update" ("Chronic Vaginitis," January–February 1988).

Printed in the United States of America on acid-free paper containing a high percentage of recycled fiber.

ISBN 0–87857–806–4 hardcover

2 4 6 8 10 9 7 5 3 1 hardcover

Notice

This book is intended as a reference volume only, not as a medical manual or guide to self-treatment. If you suspect that you have a medical problem, we urge you to seek competent medical help. Keep in mind that nutritional and health needs vary from person to person, depending on age, sex, health status, and total diet. The information here is intended to help you make informed decisions about your health, not as a substitute for any treatment that may have been prescribed by your doctor.

Contributors to the *Medical Care Yearbook*

EDITORIAL DIRECTOR: Mark Bricklin, Editor, *Prevention*® Magazine

COMPILER AND EDITOR: Sharon Stocker Ferguson, Senior Research Associate, *Prevention*® Magazine

CONTRIBUTORS: Pam Boyer, Sharon Faelten, Gloria McVeigh, Gale Maleskey, Jeff Meade, Maria Milhalik, Emrika Padus, Kerry Pechter, Porter Shimer, Maggie Spilner, Melanie Stevens, Lewis Vaughn, Susan Zarrow

EDITORIAL/PRODUCTION COORDINATOR: Jane Sherman

DESIGNER: Glen Burris

COPY EDITOR: Linda Lipkis

ASSOCIATE RESEARCH CHIEF, *PREVENTION*® MAGAZINE: Pam Boyer

ASSISTANT RESEARCH CHIEF, *PREVENTION*® MAGAZINE: Carole Piszczek

OFFICE MANAGER: Roberta Mulliner

OFFICE PERSONNEL: Deborah Maher, Kelly Trumbauer

Contents

Routine Dental X-Rays
Shouldn't Be So Routine........................ 11

No-Knife Alternative
to Hysterectomy 11

Vitamin E Protects Bypass Patients 12

Beware of Modern-Day Blood "Leeching"......... 13

Niacin Reduces Insulin Need
in Some Diabetics 14

Part II
Medical Care Frontiers

Chapter 1
Hot News on Laser Therapy.................. 15
An exciting look at the ways that dermatologists, urologists, ophthalmologists, and cosmetic surgeons are using lasers with great success, as well as a preview of the potential of lasers to zap life-threatening plaque from arteries and cancer from diseased tissues.

Chapter 2
Alternative "Medicine" for Back Pain........... 20
A review of back-care therapy highlights the latest and most successful trends in treatment, revealing why surgery has fallen out of favor. Includes a survey comparing the success rates of various practitioners.

Chapter 3
What Is Carpal Tunnel Syndrome?............. 32
Profile of a disease that often masquerades as arthritis and strikes one in ten Americans. Covers symptoms, risk factors, and treatments.

Part III
Health-Saving Advances

Part V
Better Ways to Beat Everyday Health Problems

Part VI
Women's Health Newsfront

Part VII
Men's Health Newsfront

Part IX
Children's Health Newsfront

Part X
The Big Picture in 1989

INTRODUCTION

Getting the Most out of Medical Care

Your body is the most high tech "machine" known to science. And to a large degree, *you* control the longevity and quality of the equipment. When you choose to eat plenty of fresh fruits and vegetables or make a commitment to a regular exercise program, you help keep it in the best possible condition.

But even with the best maintenance, parts sometimes break down. And that's when we depend on medicine to patch us up. We marvel at medical technology—conceived by scientists who focus their energy, intelligence, and creativity on one fundamental action: discovering new ways to heal the human body.

Prevention's Medical Care Yearbook for 1989 puts your finger on the pulse of this healing force. From the myriad of scientific data published yearly, the Yearbook presents the findings that are most important, most up-to-date, and most likely to improve your prospects for better health.

In the past, everybody knew the difference between preventive care and medical care. One you practiced in the privacy of your own home; the other you sought from your doctor when something went wrong. Physicians and patients went about their own business and rarely crossed over into the other's territory.

But times are definitely changing. Look at the Contents pages here and you'll see beans and bananas alongside the lasers and Lovastatin. No doubt, new developments in technology are still hot news, because we all may someday

benefit from state-of-the-art treatments like electrical stimulation that strengthens muscles, miniature camera "scopes" that let surgeons see inside the body (reducing the need for surgery), and x-rays that greatly reduce radiation doses. Some of these developments can turn what used to be a week's hospital visit into a day, or reduce the risk of infection to almost zero. Even traditional procedures are less invasive and more accurate than ever. And that's exciting.

At the same time, the role of diet in medical care is burgeoning. Potassium for strokes, calcium for cancer, tryptophan for high blood pressure—these and other vitamins, minerals, and amino acids are joining the ranks called medicine. That old distinction between medical care and preventive care has become shadowy at best.

A case in point: In 1989, the low-fat diet is both preventive *and* prescriptive care. Scientists report that eating less fat can help head off a host of villains: cancer, high blood pressure, obesity, and heart disease. But they've also found that a combination of a low-fat, low-cholesterol diet and blood pressure-lowering drugs can be prescribed as a medical treatment to lessen the threat of heart disease.

Another benefit: Preventive care can help optimize medical care. A well-nourished, well-exercised body has a stronger heart, a more active immune system, and denser bones. The mental outlook that accompanies fitness is bound to be brighter and more positive. Just imagine the effect such strength will have on recovery time and quality of healing.

It's exciting to live in the midst of the new alliance of medicine and prevention, and this year's *Medical Care Yearbook* shows how to take advantage of the benefits of this partnership.

Sharon Stocker Ferguson
Senior Research Associate
Prevention® Magazine

PART I: MEDICAL RESEARCH BULLETINS

HEART RESUSCITATORS NOW AVAILABLE FOR HOME USE

When a person's heart stops, every second counts. Getting the right help fast often means the difference between life and death.

Now people can have in their homes the same kind of equipment emergency medical crews use to restart a heart. Called automatic external defibrillators, these machines can possibly shock the fluttering heart of a heart attack victim back into rhythm long before paramedics arrive. This reduces the chance of permanent heart or brain damage, even death.

Because they can start the heart pumping again on its own, these devices are better than cardiopulmonary resuscitation, which simply maintains breathing for the victim.

"It's practically a fail-safe system," says Richard Cummins, M.D., an associate professor of medicine at the University of Washington. "The machine monitors the heart, recognizes a fibrillating pattern, and delivers a shock that stimulates a more normal pattern."

About the size of a child's lunch box and powered by batteries, the devices are available nationwide, by prescription, to high-risk heart patients. Some health insurance companies will help cover costs.

TRIPLE-CHECK PAP SMEARS

Women have been told for years that a Pap smear will tell them when they have cancer and when they don't. But what they don't know could kill them.

Doctors have known for years that the test—one of the most commonly performed—is also one of the most inaccurate. It has a 20 percent false-negative rate, according to the American College of Obstetricians and Gynecologists. It fails to detect about one out of five cell abnormalities.

About half of these false-negatives are due to the doctor's cell-sampling techniques. The others are due to misinterpretation of the cells during laboratory analysis.

To improve the accuracy of your test results, Robert Hutter, M.D., chairman of the American Cancer Society's National Advisory Committee on Cancer Prevention and Detection says that you should ask your gynecologist these questions: Where is my Pap smear going to be sent? Is it a licensed and accredited laboratory? Will a pathologist check it if results are abnormal? Does the laboratory provide a full written report?

And to make sure your doctor has taken an adequate cell sample, ask him or her if the lab reports poor samples as "inadequate for evaluation" or simply as "negative."

The American Cancer Society recently revised its Pap smear guidelines. It now suggests that sexually active women, or those 18 years of age or older, get an annual Pap test until they get three consecutive satisfactory negative test results one year apart. After that, the test can be taken less frequently at the discretion of the doctor.

UPDATE ON BALDNESS DRUG

Hope has been running high for the Friar Tucks and Uncle Festers of the world since the discovery of minoxidil, a blood pressure drug that also encourages new growth on balding pates. But until recently, most men could expect this drug to stimulate little more than fuzz.

Now, though, minoxidil may be getting a boost from another drug, tretinoin, a topical form of vitamin A used to treat acne.

Researchers in New Orleans found that 66 percent of the bald men who used both drugs had hair regrowth resembling their normal hair. Using either drug alone, up to one-half of the men had some hair regrowth.

Minoxidil stimulates blood flow and production of new cells in the scalp. Tretinoin causes new blood vessels to form and helps skin shed its dead upper layers. Together they "may be more effective as promoters of new hair growth in individuals with [baldness]," say the researchers (*Journal of the American Academy of Dermatology*).

POSTURAL THERAPY RELIEVES PELVIC PAIN

Can a slumping pose make your innards hurt? It's pretty common knowledge that poor posture can cause back pain. Now a study from the University of Tennessee shows that it might be a cause of pelvic pain as well.

After a thorough physical examination, 75 women with

pelvic pain were referred for physical therapy. More than two-thirds were found to have faulty posture.

"Certain postures—lordosis [swayback] and kyphosis [humpback]—are of particular concern when dealing with pelvic pain," says physical therapist Patricia M. King. "These postures lead to an imbalance of muscle strength in the back and abdomen. The abdomen becomes stretched while the back is strained."

The women learned exercises aimed at stretching tight back muscles and strengthening weak abdominal muscles. They were taught good posture and received hot packs, massage, and/or ultrasound therapy as needed. Of 59 women who stuck with the program, 39 had significant relief from pelvic pain and 12 had complete relief.

"Some women have more than one cause of pelvic pain," says Frank W. Ling, M.D., an associate professor of obstetrics and gynecology at the University of Tennessee. "Even with another condition, such as endometriosis or fibroids, bad posture is an added element of pain. When we correct the posture, alleviating that pain, the patient's overall pain is lessened."

BLOOD PRESSURE READINGS OFTEN OFF

Were you told you have high blood pressure after only one visit to the doctor's office? If so, it's possible you're being treated for a condition you don't have.

Researchers in Canada found that when a diagnosis was based on just one reading, one of every four people who appeared to have high blood pressure actually did not. "These people may have 'white-coat apprehension,'" says Nicholas Birkett, M.D., the study's main researcher. "Their blood pressure may have been higher than usual during the reading because they were nervous."

But when blood pressure was taken on two additional, separate occasions, such people were weeded out. Their blood pressure had dropped to within normal range.

To make an accurate diagnosis of mild high blood pressure, Dr. Birkett says, it's best to take three or four separate readings over as long as six months (*Canadian Medical Association Journal*).

TESTOSTERONE HELPS MENOPAUSAL WOMEN

Doctors have known for years that all women have in their blood small amounts of the male hormone testosterone. They've also known that testosterone levels drop at menopause or with removal of the ovaries.

Until recently, they had no idea what testosterone does in women. As a result, they made no attempt to replace it when levels were low. Now, though, studies by Barbara Sherwin, Ph.D., of McGill University in Montreal, show that testosterone plays a crucial role in maintaining a woman's quality of life.

She's studied women who have had their ovaries removed during a hysterectomy. When these women received a once-a-month injection of a testosterone/estrogen drug, they said they felt more energetic and were more interested in sex than when they received estrogen or a placebo only. They were much less likely to complain of feeling tired, irritable, nervous, or depressed.

"They feel better, plain and simple," Dr. Sherwin says. One concern—that testosterone might elevate blood cholesterol—proved unfounded, at least with the injectable form. And only 10 to 15 percent of the women Dr. Sherwin has treated have developed mild reversible hirsutism, or facial hair.

"Many of these women are on long-term estrogen because it protects against osteoporosis and heart disease,"

Dr. Sherwin says. "Whether they also need testosterone is an individual matter. I would say that 75 percent of the women we see are candidates for it. They may report lack of sexual interest in an otherwise good relationship, or they might be working women who are just not feeling as peppy as they'd like."

Although still not routine, this treatment is being offered by more and more gynecologists, Dr. Sherwin says.

DO-IT-YOURSELF BRAIN STIMULATION RELIEVES SEVERE PAIN

A new surgical procedure can make life worth living again for some people with chronic pain. The new technique, developed by doctors at the University of California at San Francisco, involves implanting electrodes in the area of the brain where the body's natural painkillers, called endorphins, are released. Electrical stimulation through the electrodes causes the release of these "natural opiates," easing pain, the doctors believe.

People who undergo the procedure carry a special radio transmitter, which they use to stimulate the electrodes. They also take the amino acid tryptophan, a precursor of the brain chemical serotonin. The stimulation decreases serotonin, and the extra tryptophan makes up for that loss. The procedure is a last resort for people whose pain cannot be controlled by drugs. Although it doesn't eliminate all pain, it can make a tremendous difference.

The success rate for the surgery was about 80 percent in the first 122 people to have it. The doctors attribute the success to the fact that the people were screened carefully to be sure the surgery was right for them.

NEW PROSTATE CANCER DETECTOR

A new blood test provides a simple and certain way to detect prostate disease, including cancer. The test—called prostate-specific antigen immunoassay—can detect amounts of a substance less than a billionth of a gram per milliliter of blood. It measures concentrations of a special type of protein known as prostate-specific antigen. An elevation of this protein, which is normally present in the blood in small amounts, indicates prostate disease or possibly prostate cancer.

"This is an excellent test for someone over 50 to have yearly," says Carl Killian, Ph.D., of Roswell Park Memorial Institute in Buffalo, where the test was developed. The test can also indicate if prostate cancer therapy is working or if the cancer has moved to other parts of the body. This "tumor marker" blood test is approved by the Food and Drug Administration and is commercially available to physicians.

HOW TO AVOID UNNECESSARY FOOT SURGERY

Orthopedic doctors used to think chronic heel pain was usually caused by calcium deposits called bone "spurs." Now they have found that such pain is more often the result of tiny stress fractures.

New kinds of x-rays, such as bone scans and tomogra-

phy (varying "depth" x-rays), allow doctors to examine the injured foot better and make a firm diagnosis.

This finding should help eliminate unnecessary foot surgery, says Charles Graham, M.D., of the University of Texas Health Science Center at Dallas. "We know now that bone spurs usually don't cause pain and so don't need to be removed. And for stress fractures, walking and stretching exercises and a heel pad in your shoe are all you need." Get a second opinion if your doctor suggests surgery, Dr. Graham urges.

LIGHTWEIGHT SENIORS RISK OVERDOSING

Doctors at Harvard Medical School recently found that older, underweight people frequently get prescribed drugs in too high a dose because their doctors fail to take into account their age or weight. People who weighed 110 pounds or less were at greatest risk: Their dosages were 31 to 46 percent higher than normal.

These conclusions were based on thousands of prescriptions written for three common drugs. These medications can, in large amounts, cause kidney damage, confusion, or harmful drug interactions. Dosages of drugs that are highly toxic, like cancer drugs, are always calculated by body weight, says the study's organizer, Edward W. Campion, M.D.

"There *is* room for improvement in calculating correct dosage," Dr. Campion says. "If you are very thin, it's worthwhile to remind your doctor how much you weigh."

ELECTRICAL TREATMENT STRENGTHENS WEAK BACK MUSCLES

Electricity may have the potential to heal injured back muscles, according to researchers from the Hospital for Joint Diseases Orthopedic Institute in New York City. It's known that low back pain is improved by exercises that increase back strength and endurance. But in a study of 114 healthy women, Margareta Nordin, Ph.D., associate director, and colleagues found that stimulating back muscles with electricity increased muscle strength as much as isometric exercise did. In addition, the women receiving mild electrical stimulation had more muscle endurance than those doing isometrics. Preliminary studies on patients with low back pain are showing similar results.

The treatment is meant to complement, not replace, exercise, though. "I think this will be especially beneficial to the patients who have acute and chronic back pain," says Dr. Nordin. "They can receive this treatment to strengthen back muscles so that they can begin an exercise program sooner."

The treatment is much like TENS (transcutaneous electrical nerve stimulation), which is used for pain relief, but it uses less electricity. It is not painful. Pads are placed on the muscles at each side of the lower spine, and the muscles on both sides are stimulated so that they contract and relax at the same time. That action is similar to what happens during isometric exercise.

HEART DIAGNOSIS BY TELEPHONE IS HERE

It's tough sometimes for doctors trying to diagnose their patients' irregular heartbeat. The heart may do all its fluttering and sputtering at home but refuse to act up in the doctor's office. That makes diagnosis and treatment difficult. And it may mean a problem isn't treated as promptly as it should be.

Now, though, it's possible to capture the heart's idiosyncrasies on paper, within minutes, with a device called an event transmitter and a phone call.

You put the transmitter, a box the size of a small radio, on your chest, call your medical center, identify yourself, and place the telephone mouthpiece on the unit. A machine at the other end monitors your heartbeat, creating an instant electrocardiogram. The doctor on duty can immediately interpret the results and make a diagnosis.

Pacemaker patients have been using these devices to check their hearts for more than ten years. "The ideal new user," says David R. Holmes, M.D., cardiologist at the Mayo Clinic in Rochester, Minnesota, "is the arrhythmia sufferer who has spells that are intermittent (making them hard to diagnose) and lengthy enough (10 or 15 minutes) to last through a phone call."

Patients at the Mayo Clinic take a transmitter home on loan, then pay around $30 whenever they use it.

ROUTINE DENTAL X-RAYS SHOULDN'T BE SO ROUTINE

Does your dentist routinely x-ray your teeth for hidden cavities? If so, you may be interested in this: A new study compared the effectiveness at finding cavities of a careful dental examination and bite-wing x-rays on both sides of the mouth. Only 11 percent of the patients with no clinical signs of decay showed any cavities on the x-rays, and most were superficial cavities that would not have required immediate treatment.

"Dental x-rays *do* pose a risk for cancer," says researcher George Kaugars, D.D.S., of the Medical College of Virginia in Richmond. "Even though that risk is very small, it should not be ignored."

He suggests that healthy adults with no signs of cavities get dental x-rays no more often than every 18 months.

NO-KNIFE ALTERNATIVE TO HYSTERECTOMY

A slender scope that lets doctors view and operate in the uterus without an incision could cut in half the need for hysterectomy.

The instrument, a hysteroscope, contains a miniature lens, a light source, and a passageway for surgical instruments. It's inserted through the vagina into the uterus. The lens is used to locate the problem, and various surgical instruments are used to correct the condition. A fibroid

tumor protruding into the uterine cavity, for example, can be shaved down with an electrified probe. The lining of the uterus can be cauterized using a laser.

Right now, the hysteroscope is most often used for diagnosis and biopsy, says Robert Neuwirth, M.D., director of St. Luke's/Roosevelt Hospital Department of Gynecology in New York City. "But as more and more doctors learn to use it for surgery, we expect it to become a good alternative to diagnostic dilatation and curettage [D and C] and hysterectomy."

VITAMIN E PROTECTS BYPASS PATIENTS

Bypass surgery is meant to circumvent years of arterial damage caused by heart disease. But this extensive operation also *causes* some damage. It creates an excess of destructive particles called free radicals. In bypass surgery, free-radical activity can cause microscopic damage to the cells of the lungs and heart.

Researchers at the Mayo Clinic in Rochester, Minnesota, decided recently to see how vitamin E affects free-radical formation in heart bypass patients. Vitamin E is one of the most potent free-radical quenchers known.

They found that patients given 2,000 international units of vitamin E 12 hours before bypass surgery had much lower blood levels of free radicals than patients who did not get vitamin E. They also found that, in unsupplemented patients, vitamin E levels plummeted after surgery. In the patients who had received the vitamin E dose before surgery, levels remained normal.

"I'd recommend that patients receive a dose of vitamin E before heart surgery," says the study's main researcher, Nicholas Cavarocchi, M.D., now at Temple University in Philadelphia. "An adequate amount of this vitamin could help make this a safer procedure."

BEWARE OF MODERN-DAY BLOOD "LEECHING"

The way some hospital patients are treated, you might think their doctors are out for blood—literally.

Investigators from Harvard Medical School found that the average patient had blood taken slightly more often than once a day. During his stay, he lost about ¾ cup of blood for tests. The average patient in an intensive care unit had blood taken more than three times a day and was leeched of more than 3 cups. Intensive care patients who had IV tubes in their arms lost an average of 4 cups.

In many of these patients, this bloodletting caused anemia and contributed to the need for later transfusions to replace the blood, a procedure that carries its own risks.

Taking so much blood from patients simply isn't necessary, the researchers argue. Current laboratory instruments require very little blood for testing, they say, so that small specimen tubes of the size normally used for children would be sufficient. Switching to these smaller tubes would cut the blood loss by 40 to 45 percent.

The doctors also observed that various routine tests that could have been performed with just one tube of blood were ordered at different times of the day, which meant that a new tube had to be drawn for each test. Simply batching the tests would reduce blood loss the same way combining errands saves gasoline.

"A critical evaluation of test-ordering habits is important not only for the purpose of promoting cost containment and laboratory efficiency but also for reducing or eliminating the transfusions required to replace blood drawn for diagnostic tests," the doctors say.

They recommend that a daily tally of blood loss be kept for each patient and that doctors take this into consideration before ordering additional tests (*New England Journal of Medicine*).

NIACIN REDUCES INSULIN NEED IN SOME DIABETICS

New evidence from researchers in France suggests that niacinamide, a form of the B vitamin niacin, may give hope to newly diagnosed diabetics.

Type I (or juvenile) diabetes results when the beta cells of the pancreas don't function adequately. The beta cells are responsible for producing insulin, the hormone that helps your body use glucose, the basic food of cells.

In a recent study, French researchers gave either niacinamide or a placebo (a harmless, inactive substitute) to 16 people who had just been diagnosed as having Type I diabetes. All of the people had needed insulin to control their symptoms.

After one year, three of the seven people receiving the niacinamide were in remission—they no longer needed insulin. None of the nine people in the placebo group were in remission. After three years, two of the people receiving niacinamide were still in remission.

"Complete remissions for over two years are rarely achieved in young adult patients with Type I insulin-dependent diabetes," say the researchers. "Our results and those from animal experiments indicate that, in Type I diabetes, [niacinamide] slows down destruction of beta cells and enhances their regeneration, thus extending remission time" (*Lancet*).

PART II: MEDICAL CARE FRONTIERS

CHAPTER 1

Hot News on Laser Therapy

On a scale of one to ten, the progression of laser technology is rated only four, but it has already replaced the knife in numerous procedures.

When scientists first used lasers to dissolve ruptured blood vessels in the human eye over 20 years ago, they were as excited as the frenzied photons they had finally harnessed. Here was a whole new edge in medicine—not just a bloodless scalpel of incredible precision but also a cellular soldering gun and possibly even a tissue "regenerator," depending on the type and intensity of light waves generated.

Have lasers lived up to these high hopes? How exactly do they work? And in what ways are they ready *now* to shine their healing lights on you?

These questions were posed to George M. Bohigian, M.D., associate clinical professor of ophthalmology at the University of Washington School of Medicine. In addition to using laser therapy in his private practice as an ophthalmologist for over 15 years, Dr. Bohigian reviewed the use of lasers in other specialties as chairman of the American Medical Association's Council on Scientific Affairs.

Lasers are currently enjoying their greatest successes in procedures demanding great delicacy—gynecology, cosmetic surgeries, tumor removals, and surgeries of the eye, Dr. Bohigian says. Many other applications, however, are being investigated—everything from clearing arteries of life-threatening plaque to vaporizing cancer cells. "On a scale of one to ten, I'd say we've reached only about a four in realizing the full medical potential of lasers in the future," Dr. Bohigian says.

Like Hulk Hogan in Heels

And how exactly do lasers work?

Laser is an acronym for *l*ight *a*mplification by *s*timulated *e*mission of *r*adiation, but if those words beam right by you, don't feel bad.

"I tell people to think of lasers as someone very large in a pair of very narrow high heels," Dr. Bohigian explains. "Lots of energy, in the form of light, gets directed into a very narrow focus. The burning ray of light you create with a magnifying glass and the sun is a crude form of laser."

Crude indeed, because lasers used for medical purposes not only shine much hotter but can be focused into a beam less than a millionth of a millimeter in width. That's small enough, theoretically, to do corrective surgery on malformed genes! Lasers also can be controlled to emit bursts lasting only billionths of a second—crucial in surgeries demanding that the laser's heat be confined to microscopically small areas.

"The CO_2 laser can generate heat so intense that tissue under target—cancer cells, for example—turns instantaneously to vapor," Dr. Bohigian says.

Tissue immediately adjacent to this obliteration merely gets seared (cauterized), however, which is a huge advantage in that the surgeon can work virtually blood free. "In surgeries demanding great precision, this is a godsend," Dr. Bohigian says. "Not only does the surgeon have an instrument of incredible accuracy, he has an amazingly clear field in which to use it. Risks of infection are also greatly minimized because incisions can be made with tissue never actually being touched."

Different Speeds for Different Needs

But lasers can do more than just cut. Lower their intensity a notch and tissue is not evaporated but only coagulated, much like the white of an egg when it's fried. Lower the intensity one more notch and you get merely a warming effect known as photodisruption, a process that subtly alters a tissue's molecular structure.

"Coagulation is useful in conditions such as bleeding ulcers and other internal hemorrhaging, where ruptured blood vessels must be not so much destroyed as rendered inactive," Dr. Bohigian explains. "We use this technique to stop bleeding in the eye, which is a common and potentially serious consequence of diabetic retinopathy."

As for photodisruption, it's one of "the more investigational areas of laser therapy," Dr. Bohigian says, but it's exciting nonetheless. The procedure has been shown to encourage not only tissue healing but also tissue destruction when used in conjunction with certain photosensitive drugs. "This is one of the more promising areas of cancer research," says Dr. Bohigian. Cancer cells are impregnated with chemicals that cause the cells to self-destruct when exposed to the laser's light.

What's Ready Now

Experimental areas aside, what forms of laser therapy are ready and available now?

"Lasers are being used most widely in the fields of ophthalmology, dermatology, urology, and cosmetic surgery," says Dr. Bohigian. "The precision, fast healing, and low risk of infection with lasers make them especially suited for these specialties. Some procedures are now routine, in fact, that in the past weren't even possible."

In ophthalmology, for example, many of the procedures used to treat diabetic retinopathy, cataracts, and glaucoma were not possible as recently as ten years ago. Dermatology and cosmetic surgery have also gained greatly from laser therapy. In dermatology, lasers are removing everything from skin tags to genital warts with unprecedented ease, while cosmetic surgeons are erasing acne scars, port-

wine stains, spider veins, age spots, freckles, tattoos, and even facial wrinkles.

And in urology . . . well, grit your teeth if you must, but the boon here has been laser therapy via flexible glass tubing (about the thickness of a human hair) fed into internal territory by way of the urethra. Cancer of the bladder has been the primary target.

Risks Not So Risky

But with these miraculous benefits of lasers must come at least some garden-variety risks, right?

"No more so than with more conventional therapies if proper precautions are taken by the laser therapist," Dr. Bohigian says. "Risks may even be less with many laser procedures because less anesthesia is needed, risks of infection are reduced, and greater precision is possible."

Precautions to be observed by the laser-wielding therapist, Dr. Bohigian says, should include protection of body areas adjacent to the laser's focus, adequate evacuation of fumes created by a laser's tissue-vaporizing action, and selection of nonflammable general anesthetic in cases where a laser is being used. There can be a very real risk of "patient fire" if this precaution is not taken, Dr. Bohigian says.

Finding a Surgeon

So how do you know if there's a laser therapy available for a problem you have, and how do you go about finding a laser surgeon competent to treat that problem?

One way is to contact the American Society for Laser Medicine and Surgery (813 Second Street, Suite 200, Wausau, WI 54401) and explain your condition. If laser therapy seems promising, you'll be provided with a list of qualified laser surgeons in your area.

Or, as Dr. Bohigian recommends, you can call your local county or state medical society. Make sure to ask for surgeons who have been "board-certified," Dr. Bohigian says, because this assures you that they've passed appropriate tests of competence. It's advisable to lean toward a surgeon

who is affiliated with a respectable university hospital as well. ("Good universities value their good reputations," Dr. Bohigian says.) It's probably a good idea to ask a prospective surgeon about his experience, too. If you can also find some references—patients who can vouch for a surgeon's expertise personally—you're one step closer to a wise choice, according to Dr. Bohigian.

A Look to the Future

If, as Dr. Bohigian says, we've reached only about a four out of ten in realizing the full potential of lasers in medicine, what might those other six points bring?

Already lasers have achieved encouraging results in clearing arteries of life-threatening plaque. They're also showing promise in "welding" arteries in surgeries such as the coronary bypass, where vessels must be replaced or repaired. Scientists have high hopes, too, for employing lasers in diagnostic roles where lasers, by way of catheters, will be able to view internal organs in 3-D.

Perhaps most intriguing, however, is the potential of lasers in the fight against cancer. With lung cancer, for example, the hope is to arrest malignancies in their early stages, possibly by directing laser beams at cancerous tissue through catheters, in much the same way they're being aimed at arterial plaque.

Even grander is the scheme of one day being able to perform corrective surgery on defective genes that may be responsible for the development of disease in the first place.

How's that for beating the enemy to the punch?

CHAPTER 2

Alternative "Medicine" for Back Pain

Sufferers have found long-term relief from physiatrists and yoga instructors.

On November 9, 1986, back care was catapulted forward—or backward—five years, depending on your point of view. On that day, Joe Montana, the quarterback of the San Francisco 49ers, returned to the football field just eight weeks after extensive surgery to repair a ruptured disk, one of the cartilaginous shock absorbers between the vertebrae in his back. Montana's "slipped disk" was only part of his problem. He also suffered from spinal stenosis, a congenital condition in which the bony spaces through his vertebrae were too small for the nerves radiating from his spinal column. As a result, Montana's ruptured disks caused unusually severe pain.

Many experts shook their heads as Arthur White, M.D., and a team of back surgeons operated on Montana in September of 1986. Despite the fact that some 200,000 North Americans still have back surgery every year, over the last decade the scalpel has been largely discredited as a back-care tool. Back surgery is invasive and very expensive, and it provides lasting relief from low back pain in less than one-third of all cases. The pundits predicted that Joe would be out for the season—and would probably never play football again. But on that second Sunday in November, Joe Montana did the impossible. He returned to the playing field and threw three touchdown passes to lead the 49ers to victory over the St. Louis Cardinals—a medical miracle.

The experts, including Montana's own surgeon, warned that Joe's back was "a special case," and that surgery should be considered only as a last resort for back prob-

lems. But to no avail. Thousands of people with low back pain hobbled to surgeons, demanding that they perform a "Montana."

To Ann Borgenicht, a 35-year-old San Francisco nurse, "Montana" is the state east of Idaho. Her back problem was never the subject of sports-page hand-wringing, but it was the kind that hundreds of thousands of people suffer each year. Without any history of back problems, one day she bent over and something snapped. "The pain was so intense, I couldn't stand it," she recalls. "I had to have friends drive me to my appointments while I lay in pain on the back seat." Surgery was out of the question: Borgenicht wouldn't consider it. Instead, she spent five months shuttling among orthopedists, chiropractors, physical therapists, acupuncturists, and a neurologist—until she found a bodywork therapist who specialized in exercise rehabilitation. Six weeks of gentle, self-directed movement put her on the road to recovery.

It would be difficult to find another condition that responds to two more opposite therapeutic approaches. The back is truly a mystery.

One of the few certainties about the back is that many different conditions can make it hurt. Another is that never before have there been as many back-care practitioners, programs, and products—everything from masseurs to surgeons; yoga to rowing machines; videos to whirlpool baths. Most back sufferers quickly become as exasperated about where to turn for help as they are tortured by pain. All back-care therapies are controversial. Practitioners in every specialty argue that their approach is the way to go. Few really understand how their methods compare with the competition. Comparison is vital because at some point in their lives, four out of five North Americans experience back pain severe enough to disrupt their lives, and millions have chronically bad backs. Authorities estimate that back care is now a $23-billion-a-year industry.

Looking Back

The quick fix remains elusive in the world of back treatment, but today sufferers stand a better chance of returning

to pain-free lives than ever before. We are now in the third decade of what some call the Back-Care Revolution.

Through the 1960s, chronic back problems were treated almost exclusively by physicians, who prescribed some combination of bed rest, drugs, and surgery. These methods sometimes worked, but at least half the time they didn't. In fact, they often made people feel worse. As back sufferers—and their physicians—realized that the orthodox approach wasn't the answer, back-care philosophy began to change profoundly.

Extended use of painkilling drugs came in for a good deal of criticism. Pain medication and muscle relaxants often mask underlying problems and make evaluation and treatment more difficult. Today, most physicans prescribe pain medication more sparingly, usually only during acute episodes of severe back pain.

Surgery also fell into disfavor. "Surgery is almost never necessary," says Joe Montana's surgeon. Dr. White, one of the nation's leading back specialists, says that surgery—now among the least popular forms of back therapy—deserves its bad reputation. "Surgeons have blinders on," he says. "All they know is surgery." Strong words for the man who put one of the finest quarterbacks in history under the knife. But Dr. White says that in Montana's case, there was no alternative. "Surgery is indicated if the pain does not respond to other treatments and if it's complicated by progressive loss of nerve function. Montana had had disk problems before, and nothing gave him adequate relief. After his injury, he was in so much pain he couldn't walk. Given his history, his spinal stenosis, and the progressive nerve loss he was suffering, nobody who knows anything about the spine would have objected to surgery."

But Dr. White is quick to point to the down side of Joe Montana's happy ending—more requests for back surgery. "I've received many requests to perform operations like Montana's from people who don't realize that their back problems are totally different. Montana's case was 1 in 100. We've always done far too much back surgery in this country. Back surgery is less popular than ever, yet we still do twice as much per capita as in England and many other countries."

During the 1950s and 1960s, the frequent failure of orthodox back care drove millions of Americans to their first encounter with an alternative healing art, namely chiropractic. Based on spinal manipulation, chiropractic had been around for decades. At the time, most physicians viewed it about as sympathetically as witchcraft. Thirty years ago, physicians often warned that to consult a chiropractor was to risk being "crippled for life."

But many back sufferers found relief through chiropractic, and by the late 1970s, so many physicians were referring back patients to chiropractors that the American Medical Association (AMA)—which had held it in contempt for decades—removed all objections to referring back problems to chiropractors. It was a humbling moment for the AMA, one that opened doors to the many alternative healing arts flourishing today.

The other major development in the 1970s was the realization that many back problems are linked to poor posture, obesity, sedentary lifestyle, improper lifting, and poor physical conditioning. Suddenly back sufferers were exhorted to get involved in their own treatment through exercise, weight loss, and lifestyle adjustments.

This development signaled a growing awareness of why so many people endure back pain in the first place. The human back is an engineering disaster. Walking upright forces the lower back to support much of the body's weight, something it is poorly equipped to do. And when we're not walking, we're often sitting in chairs that provide little or no lower back support. The result is our epidemic of disk problems.

Trauma or the accumulated stress of bad posture or extra weight causes the sensitive disks to rupture. The inner pulp leaks out and presses on the spinal nerves, causing pain. A less severe—but still painful—variation occurs when the disks don't actually rupture but instead bulge at the nerve roots.

Poor posture, improper lifting, and weight problems are endemic in our culture and begin with young children. Add psychological stresses, the trauma of things like automobile accidents, and the weak abdominal and thigh muscles of an average white-collar lifestyle, and you have a

profile of many of those in the 80 percent back-sufferer majority.

But physical fitness is only part of the answer—and a controversial part at that. Consider the debate over the sit-up. Some back specialists swear by it as the path to a strong abdomen to support a weak back. Others call it dangerous, a one-way ticket to back disaster.

The current consensus is that muscle tone has its place in back rehabilitation but that stretching and movement training are more important. Even superathlete Joe Montana had to learn how to bend to avoid further trouble. Each time your foot strikes the ground during a hard run, your back absorbs a force equal to four times your weight. In today's exercise-manic world of joggers, rowers, weight trainers, and aerobic dancers—many of whom took up exercise in part because of back problems—all sorts of overuse injuries have become commonplace. Particularly susceptible are the "weekend warriors," who push far beyond the limits of their conditioning. This injury epidemic has been a big factor in the popularization of less stressful conditioning activities such as swimming, walking, and low-impact aerobics.

The Dike Breaks

In the 1980s, the scope of back-care philosophy has broadened. Today, back problems are viewed as lifestyle issues, not just pathology to be cured. Information abounds. An estimated 300 books have been published on self-help for back and neck pain.

When physicians withdrew their objections to chiropractic for back care, a medical dike broke, and we've become inundated with a torrent of new back therapies. This emerging interdisciplinary field is increasingly oriented toward exercise, self-care, and encouraging back sufferers to take maximum responsibility for their recovery. But treatments vary widely, and it's not easy to select from among the bewildering variety of practitioners.

Another cornerstone of contemporary back care is the back products industry, one of the fastest-growing segments of the self-care marketplace. In 1980, there were

fewer than five lumbar support devices available to relieve low back pain. Today there are more than 100, including a dizzying array of pillows, heating and cooling devices, traction units, and ergonomic—that is, human oriented—chairs, car seat inserts, and work stations for people with bad backs.

Backsavers to the Rescue

At first glance, it looks like a furniture store filled with chairs, desks, and beds. But on closer inspection, most of the chairs look a bit unusual—and how many furniture stores sell shovels, rakes, car seat inserts, and wedge-shaped pillows? This is no ordinary furniture store. It's Back Designs, the San Francisco Bay Area's most complete back store, one of an estimated 250 to 500 such stores serving the bad backs of North America.

"I never meant to go into this business," physical therapist and Back Designs founder Eileen Vollowitz says with a laugh. "But in the early 1980s, I was specializing in back problems. I kept urging my clients to buy back-supporting chairs, and either they couldn't find them or else they bought things that were wrong for their back. The first back store had opened in Boston around then, and a group of us decided to do one here. I raised the start-up money from other practitioners three years ago, and here we are—the only back store I know of owned and operated by back-care professionals."

Vollowitz says that backs, like feet, come in many shapes and sizes, and that, like shoes, back products must be fitted individually. "Some people have flat backs and need flat support," she says. "Others have curved backs and need lumbar supports with different curvatures. Comfort is the key."

(continued)

Backsavers to the Rescue—Continued

Vollowitz welcomes the trend toward individualized back care and hopes that it reduces the faddishness of such back products as kneeling chairs. "The manufacturers say that kneeling chairs are good for any seated task, and the promotional brochures often show them being used at computer work stations. But in our experience, that isn't the case. Kneeling chairs are great for people who sit leaning forward—doing writing, drafting, drawing, reaching, dentistry, and lab work," she says. "But if you sit erect or leaning back—doing typing, computer work, telephoning, or watching TV—they usually don't provide enough support. Also, the bend in the knees makes them too cramped for tall, long-legged people. Kneeling chairs certainly have their place, but like all back products, they're not for everyone."

Although back stores have pioneered the development of back-sparing designs, the furniture industry as a whole is not far behind. "Ergonomics is all the rage now," Vollowitz says. "The Europeans developed back-supporting furnishings years ago, but until recently in the United States, fashion took precedence over function. That's starting to change now. There's no reason people should have to wait until they have back pain to invest in an ergonomic chair. Back-supportive furnishings can be preventive as well as therapeutic."

Back products can be costly, but they're more than worth their price to those with severe back pain. Office chairs run $200 to $800, chairs for home use cost about $500, car seat inserts range from $15 to $100, and support pillows cost $25 to $40.

Should back sufferers spend hundreds of dollars on special chairs if a rolled-up towel provides equal relief? "Of course not," Vollowitz says. "I'm a big believer in rolled-up towels. For some backs, they're great, but for others, they don't work. Use whatever works for you—whatever relieves your pain and keeps you pain-free."

No Research

Unfortunately, today's freedom to choose among an unprecedented number of back-care therapies has itself become a form of tyranny. Selecting the right practitioner, chair, or exercise program is essential but chancy. Virtually no comparative, controlled clinical research has been conducted on back therapies or products, and the "experts" often disagree.

Arthur C. Klein, a New York market researcher, learned this the hard way—and we're all better off because of it. After months of excruciating low back pain and frustrating, unproductive experiences with several back specialists, Klein and his wife, science writer Dava Sobel, took matters into their own hands.

They placed ads in national magazines, asking back sufferers to complete a detailed questionnaire on their back-care experiences. Almost 500 people with hard-core bad backs responded. The Klein/Sobel survey does not pretend to be statistically valid; the respondents were self-selected, and their answers were impressionistic, not standardized.

Nonetheless, the survey, published in the book *Backache Relief,* is fascinating. It's the first attempt to compare the various forms of back care—and it shatters myths on every page.

Among nine back practitioners commonly consulted for chronic pain, respondents had the best success with yoga teachers. Nearly everyone who tried individually designed yoga exercises reported long-term relief. And yoga was the *only* therapy that none of the respondents found ineffective or counterproductive.

The next-best track record belongs to a little-known medical specialty, physiatry. Physiatrists are M.D.'s who specialize in musculoskeletal rehabilitation—from everyday aches and pains to catastrophic accidents. Respondents who consulted physiatrists reported long-term relief 86 percent of the time. Physical therapists were moderately successful, but they made 10 percent of respondents feel worse. Acupuncturists and chiropractors fell in the middle range, garnering both rave reviews and criticism.

Neurologists earned by far the worst record. They prescribed more drugs than any other doctors, were ineffective 76 percent of the time, and made 16 percent of their patients worse. Orthopedists, internists, neurosurgeons, and family practitioners did not fare much better.

But before you stop reading and flip to the yellow pages listings under Yoga, look at the table "The Ratings" below. *Every* form of back therapy helped at least some respon-

The Ratings

The following table, from the book *Backache Relief*, by Arthur C. Klein and Dava Sobel, shows how 492 chronic back pain sufferers rated their practitioners.

Since the participants were self-selected from ads in national magazines, their responses are impressionistic. However, the Klein/Sobel survey is the first systematic attempt at comparing back care specialists, and the results, while by no means definitive, are intriguing.

	Moderate to Dramatic Long-Term Relief (%)	Temporary Relief Only (%)	No Relief (%)	Made Person Feel Worse (%)
Yoga instructors	96	4	0	0
Physiatrists	86	0	7	7
Physical therapists	65	8	17	10
Acupuncturists	36	32	28	4
Chiropractors	28	28	33	11
Orthopedists	23	9	61	7
Neurosurgeons	26	8	51	15
Family Practitioners/ Internists	20	14	54	12
Neurologists	4	4	76	16

dents achieve moderate to dramatic long-term relief. Then reflect on survey researcher Klein's personal experience. His chronic, debilitating pain was finally diagnosed as a congenital neuromuscular disorder. He was cured by—you guessed it—a neurosurgeon.

How to Handle *Your* Problem

Top back specialists agree that every back problem is different and should be treated with an individualized approach. But no matter which method or combination of therapies you choose, remember that *you* are the ultimate solution. Informed self-care should be the goal of all back sufferers. Short of an emergency, these steps should significantly increase your chances of success.

Recognize your problem. "I denied my back pain for about five months—until it was unbearable," Ann Borgenicht recalls. "I kept thinking it would go away, that I'd be back on my feet the next morning." Denial is dangerous. It can lead to more severe injury and necessitate more extensive therapy. If you experience significant back or neck pain, or any numbness in a foot, leg, arm, or hand, see a physician for evaluation.

Consult your physician. Back pain can be caused by everything from kidney stones to heart problems. Most back specialists agree that only a physician is qualified to rule out the myriad of diseases that may produce back pain.

Don't let anyone talk you out of it. With the exception of physiatrists, physicians are notorious for dismissing back pain as imaginary, neurotic, or evidence of malingering. Chiropractors are popular, despite their mediocre showing in the Klein/Sobel survey, in part because they always take reports of back pain seriously.

Don't let anyone talk you into anything. Since almost everyone has a bad-back story, those with unresolved back pain inevitably become the targets of well-meaning but often overly insistent friends and relatives who urge them to try the orthopedist, acupuncturist, kneeling chair, or YMCA video that cured them. Thank these good-hearted souls, then think long and hard before taking their advice.

Remember, every back-care specialist in the Klein/Sobel survey helped some people—and every specialist (except yoga instructors) hurt others. Only you can figure out what your back needs.

Diagnose your diagnosis. Most respondents in the Klein/Sobel study received two or more completely different diagnoses. Despite the trend toward interdisciplinary back care, many practitioners of every therapeutic stripe continue to sell all back problems in terms of their own narrow specialties. Some chiropractors blame all back pain on spinal misalignment. Some acupuncturists see blocked vital energy in every back twinge. And surgeons often recommend surgery. Never consent to surgery without getting a few opinions from nonsurgeons. And don't be fooled by a diagnosis that sounds so specific you figure it must be right. Klein and Sobel found that the specificity of a diagnosis had no bearing on speed of recovery.

Avoid dogmatism. Steer clear of practitioners who dismiss every other form of back therapy as useless. Any back specialist can cite cases which "prove" that competing therapies don't work. But in back care, therapeutic rigidity is the path to failure. Look for practitioners who favor a team approach based on supporting your own self-care.

Ask practitioners about their strengths and weaknesses. Good therapists freely acknowledge the kinds of back problems they have had the most—and least—success treating. Since no one helps everyone, beware of any practitioner whose track record sounds too good to be true. It probably is.

Exercise, exercise, exercise. Extended bed rest, once considered a nearly universal solution for severe back pain, is now generally regarded as one of the worst things for a bad back. Bed rest and pain medications are often necessary for a few days, but one of the few points of agreement among all back-care specialists is that rehabilitative movement should begin as soon as the acute pain has subsided. But don't overdo it. In fact, don't do *anything* that causes pain. The old saw, "No pain, no gain," is ridiculous. Recommended exercises for back rehabilitation include walking, gentle yoga stretches, and swimming (but not the breaststroke, which may strain the back).

Ann Borgenicht's return to back health was helped by San Rafael, California, exercise therapist Meg Stern, an early advocate of low-stress exercises, which now enjoy growing acceptance as essential to individualized self-care programs. Stern advises her clients to "move the easiest way possible and avoid anything that hurts." By building on slow, gentle, individualized exercises and deep breathing techniques, her clients gradually stretch, strengthen, and tone the muscles that help support the lower back. Similar low-stress exercises are now available on videocassette.

Buy carefully. Since each bad back must be treated individually, no back product—pillow, chair, car seat, or whatever—is right for everyone. Don't judge a product simply by its description in a catalog or how it feels in a store. Test it for a few days. A product that fits you should feel right immediately and cause no aching, stiffness, or movement problems after extended use. Reputable back products dealers allow unconditional exchanges for a week to ten days after purchase. Don't buy from those who don't.

Hang in there. No responsible back-care specialist can predict when you'll return to normal. You may have to try several practitioners, programs, and products before you find the combination that works for you. Don't give up. "Curing a bad back means moving and living in a whole new way," Stern says. This may seem daunting, but with informed self-care and some combination of the approaches now available, most people with disabling back problems ultimately recover and live active, pain-free lives.

CHAPTER 3

What Is Carpal Tunnel Syndrome?

Often mistaken for arthritis, this disease can cripple your wrist if left untreated.

A simple flick of the wrist can accomplish a wide variety of everyday tasks—from opening a door to operating a hand-held can opener. But for those who suffer from carpal tunnel syndrome (CTS), the simplest wrist-twisting motion can trigger a burning pain. An estimated one in ten Americans will develop CTS—a numbing condition that can become permanently debilitating.

Carpal tunnel syndrome occurs when the tendons, bones, or ligaments in the wrist press against the median nerve, short-circuiting it. Ordinarily, the bones and ligaments form a protective sheath, or "tunnel," around the nerve and tendons. The median nerve is the major pathway for nerve impulses traveling from the spinal cord, down the arm, through the wrist and palm into the fingers. It supplies most of the sensation to the hand as well as most of the muscle power to the thumb.

"The median nerve is like a soft rubber pipe, with neurotransmitters flowing down the pipe and an electrical current traveling on the surface of it," says Colin Hall, M.D., a University of North Carolina neurologist. "In carpal tunnel syndrome, it's as if you laid a 2-by-4 down on top of the pipe and hampered that flow."

Intermittent numbness, pain, weakness, and a tingling or pins-and-needles sensation in the thumb, index finger, and middle finger are the first clues of CTS. These symptoms tend to be more noticeable at night. If untreated, the pain can radiate to the elbow, upper arm, and even the

shoulder. Eventually, the flow of nutrients to the nerve may be choked off and nerve impulses short-circuited. This can cause nerves of the thumb, index, and middle finger to "starve" and the thumb muscles to atrophy. Some people lose the use of their hands entirely.

That's why it's important to recognize and treat the symptoms early, before damage occurs. If you notice any of the symptoms, consult your physician. Self-diagnosis can be difficult because CTS can masquerade as a twinge of arthritis.

The standard medical test for CTS is electromyography. This involves sending an electric charge through electrodes on the skin. The test causes a brief tingling, but it's the best way to find out if the nerves of the wrist are intact and carrying normal electrical impulses.

Nobody knows exactly what causes CTS, but it seems to go hand in hand with jobs that require repetitious manual motions.

"There's tremendous evidence that carpal tunnel syndrome is work related," says Peter C. Amadio, M.D., of the Mayo Clinic in Rochester, Minnesota. "How else could you explain the fact that the people who debone meat in one particular meat-packing plant have a 20 percent surgery rate for CTS, while only 5 percent of their co-workers in nonboning activities require surgery?"

According to government reports, 23,000 workers suffer from the symptoms of this syndrome each year. That includes meat cutters, data processors, cashiers, assembly-line workers, pneumatic-hammer workers, and truck drivers (who keep their hands on the wheel for long stretches). Homemakers and weekend do-it-yourselfers may face similar "occupational hazards." Wringing wet laundry and installing insulation with a staple gun have been linked to CTS attacks.

Besides work, there are other contributing factors. Women are twice as likely to be struck by CTS as men. This may be because their wrists—and, consequently, their carpal "tunnels"—are narrower than men's. Pregnant women are especially prone, possibly due to fluid retention. Diabetes, arthritis, and menopause also increase a person's risk of CTS. Plus, a few arcane disorders like de

Quervain's disease (a problem affecting the tendons), acromegaly (an abnormal growth of the bones in middle age), and myxedema (a thyroid condition) may contribute to CTS.

Some people believe that CTS is a "threshold" disorder—one that develops when several predisposing factors occur simultaneously.

"It's like a bucket of water," says Glenda Key, a physical therapy consultant in Minneapolis. "We all start with a certain amount of 'water,' and when we add those other factors the bucket sometimes overflows."

Choosing Therapies

Sometimes the symptoms are mild: They come and go and are never troubling enough to demand professional care. At the other extreme, the condition can become so severe it seriously threatens mobility. Most CTS sufferers, however, find themselves somewhere in between. Their symptoms are annoying but not disabling. Caught in medical limbo, they're often forced to choose among a confusing array of treatment options.

Physical therapy is an effective, inexpensive treatment for mild to moderate CTS. In some cases, people have found symptom relief just by learning to use their hands in ways that don't put pressure on their median nerve. Just as longshoremen can learn how to lift without straining their backs, assembly-line workers can learn how to do repetitive-motion jobs without injuring their wrists. In fact, Key claims that physical therapy has reduced the incidence of CTS by as much as 94 percent among the factory workers she counsels.

"Our focus is on teaching people how to use their hands in a safer, easier, more comfortable way," says Key. "Most people are never really trained how to do their job right. They usually learn from the person working next to them. But we start by showing people how to do their job right, and only a minimal modification is usually needed. We even show people how to brush their hair or how to place plates in the cupboard. We call that 'worker's wisdom.' "

Another conservative approach to CTS is simply to im-

mobilize the wrist with a forearm splint, allowing the fingers to wriggle freely while giving the wrist a chance to heal. Some people wear the splint at night, when CTS symptoms tend to worsen. In some cases, a splint relieves pain within 24 hours.

The trouble is, "a splint itself can put pressure on the wrist," says Key. "We sometimes fit people with a splint on the top side of their hand. This doesn't press on their wrist; it just serves to remind them not to use their wrist in certain ways. It's like training wheels." When a splint doesn't work, doctors usually recommend steroid treatment—that is, an injection of cortisone directly into the wrist. This reduces swelling around the nerve and relieves pressure. Cortisone can reduce inflammation and pain within a couple of hours. It seems to work best when the person has had symptoms for just a short time. According to one neurosurgeon, eight out of ten people who receive steroid injections get significant relief. Steroids provide lasting relief in some CTS patients whose hand muscles and nerves are still healthy.

But cortisone becomes less effective after a few injections. That limits its use, and CTS symptoms often do recur. Also, there's a risk, though slim, that the doctor will pierce the median nerve or one of its branches with the hypodermic needle. Some doctors prescribe a nonsteroidal anti-inflammatory medication, such as Motrin, as a safer alternative to cortisone.

In recent years, vitamin B_6 supplementation has been widely publicized as a treatment for CTS. The leading champion of B_6 therapy in the United States is John M. Ellis, M.D., a physician practicing in Mount Pleasant, Texas. Dr. Ellis believes that a B_6 deficiency can bring on CTS symptoms. And he claims to have cured many of his CTS patients with B_6 doses as high as 100 times the Recommended Dietary Allowance.

The vitamin, says Dr. Ellis, "works by improving the function of the synovium, the sheath that surrounds the tendons." He routinely prescribes B_6 to pregnant women, both to reduce their tendency to retain fluids and to prevent CTS symptoms.

Over a period of seven years, Dr. Ellis and colleagues

treated 35 people who suffered from CTS symptoms and who also scored very low on a test for vitamin B_6 levels in the blood. Generally, the lower their B_6 level, the worse their CTS symptoms, he says. Within a month after taking between 100 and 200 milligrams of B_6 a day, these patients showed healthy levels of the vitamin. And after 12 weeks, their clinical symptoms improved or vanished, Dr. Ellis says.

If there's a scarcity of doctors who believe in B_6 as a treatment for CTS, it's mainly for lack of convincing proof. No research team has yet conducted a well-controlled study testing the effectiveness of vitamin B_6. Most doctors shrug their shoulders about B_6, saying that the jury is still out. Plus, reports linking nerve damage to high intakes of vitamin B_6 have many physicians worried. Self-medicating with large amounts of this vitamin is ill-advised. Talk with your physician.

Hand surgery is the last resort for CTS sufferers. When nothing else helps, when the problem has lasted for several years, and when irreversible damage to the muscles and nerves of the hand seems imminent, most doctors say, "Operate."

"I do surgery on people who have tried everything but aren't getting better," says Stephen Cash, M.D., of Jefferson Medical College in Philadelphia. "I also operate on people who have advanced cases, where the disease is starting to affect the muscles of the thumb. We do an electromyelogram test, and if the test shows that the thumb muscle is deteriorating, I recommend surgery."

In most cases, hand surgeons say, the operation can be done on an outpatient basis with local anesthesia. The surgery involves cutting the ligament to free the underlying nerve from any adhesions. Up to 90 percent of patients can expect improvement. Pain usually subsides within 12 to 48 hours. After surgery, the hand has to be fully bandaged for two weeks and shouldn't be used for heavy work for four to six weeks.

As operations go, carpal tunnel surgery is fairly routine. But keep in mind that surgery cannot guarantee revival of atrophied muscles or restore lost nerve function.

Before opting for surgery, consider all your treatment

options. Become conscious of the tasks you perform with your hands. If your job is a contributing factor, find out if you can rotate to jobs that place less strain on your wrists. If you can't, ask a physical therapist to show you how to use your hands in ways that don't aggravate the median nerve. Remember, any activity, from knitting to playing cards to using a jackhammer, can cause CTS. But *how* you do what you do can keep the problem under control.

CHAPTER 4

Cut the Fat and Clear Your Arteries

Can diet reverse the damage of heart disease? Breakthrough research says yes.

"This is one of the greatest landmark studies in medical history."

"This new study and future studies like it will rock the medical profession on its heels."

"This research will forever change the way this terrible disease is viewed and treated around the world."

Thus spoke sober-minded scientists who probably couldn't have been more enthusiastic if they had been talking about a cure for cancer or AIDS. What they were beaming about was the first hard evidence of its kind to show something that many cardiologists say is impossible: *reversing* atherosclerosis. Not just preventing or stopping it, but actually undoing the damage.

Picture this: Like ice building up in plumbing on a cold

day, cholesterol-laden lumps may be lining your arteries, slowly choking off the flow of blood. This, your doctor tells you, is atherosclerosis, or hardening of the arteries, the widespread symptom that's the main cause of heart disease. The lumps are lesions—ominous areas of blood vessel damage. And as they typically do in millions of people, the lesions grow relentlessly, nudging you slowly toward doom.

Then something odd happens, something almost unheard of: The lesions start to get smaller. Something puts the damage in reverse!

Evidence for this kind of reversal (or regression, as scientists call it) is precisely what all the fuss is about. Researchers say that in the new study, they used x-rays of blood vessels and strict scientific controls to demonstrate—better than in any previous research—that it's possible to make the artery-clogging lumps disappear.

What forced these dramatic changes in the arteries was the lowering of cholesterol in the blood through drugs and diet. And this news has sparked high hopes that diet alone may be able to literally clear your arteries—not just of cholesterol but also of the life-threatening roadblocks it helps cause.

In the milestone study, researchers from the University of Southern California School of Medicine tested and monitored 162 men with atherosclerosis who had previously undergone bypass surgery. The investigators first took angiograms (artery x-rays) of the men's diseased blood vessels to gauge the size of the damaged areas. Then they put half the men on a low-fat diet plus two cholesterol-lowering drugs and the other half on another low-fat diet plus a placebo (an inactive drug lookalike). Every patient's diet was monitored with a computerized analysis, and they did not smoke. After two years, the researchers took angiograms again of the same blood vessels and compared them with the earlier x-rays.

Contrary to conventional wisdom, the before-and-after angiograms showed clearly that dramatic changes had been wrought in the diseased arteries.

The researchers report that in over 16 percent of the drug-plus-diet group, the artery lesions got smaller. And,

perhaps just as important, in 45 percent of this group, the lesions remained unchanged—meaning that the seemingly unstoppable march of atherosclerosis had been halted.

Even in the group on the low-fat diet without drugs there were encouraging signs: 36.6 percent had unchanged lesions, and 2.4 percent had lesions that shrank *(Journal of the American Medical Association).*

"This study demonstrates that we now have the wherewithal to turn heart disease around in its early stages," says David H. Blankenhorn, M.D., chief investigator of the study. "Years ago, scientists and physicians watched with satisfaction as a newfound treatment melted away the early lesions of tuberculosis and stopped the spread of the disease in the lungs. And now we can watch again as a cholesterol-lowering treatment stops the spread of the lesions of atherosclerosis."

The Power of Diet

So just how potent were the low-fat diets alone in stalling or reversing artery damage?

"Unfortunately, our data can't tell us the relative importance of drugs and diet in affecting artery lesions," Dr. Blankenhorn says, "but clearly diet had an effect. We can, however, infer from our study that if people with atherosclerosis eat a low-fat, low-cholesterol diet (and don't smoke or have high blood pressure), at least 39 percent of them will have stable lesions—that is, their atherosclerosis damage will either diminish or stop progressing."

William Castelli, M.D., director of the renowned Framingham Heart Study, says that the case for the "regression diet" is very strong: "Dr. Blankenhorn's study and a lot of other research from around the world suggests that regression happens when you lower cholesterol in the blood—regardless of whether you do that with drugs or diet. So I think that in some people, diet alone can lower cholesterol enough to reverse the lesions of atherosclerosis."

That something as safe and simple as diet can reverse

the seemingly irreversible still has to be scientifically confirmed, which very well could happen soon since there are at least 20 regression studies going on worldwide. In the meantime, we already have several clues to the possible makeup of a regression diet.

In Dr. Blankenhorn's study, the diet associated with the biggest impact on lesions (the drug-group diet) contains about half as much fat as the typical American diet. Twenty-two percent of its calories come from fat (10 percent as polyunsaturated, 5 percent as saturated fat, and the rest as monounsaturated). And it limits cholesterol intake to less than 125 milligrams per day (about the amount in a roasted drumstick).

The diet responsible for the less dramatic but still impressive effect on lesions (placebo-group diet) is not as stringent—26 percent of total calories from fat (10 percent as polyunsaturated, 5 percent as saturated, and the rest as monounsaturated), with less than 250 milligrams of cholesterol per day. This eating plan is only a step away from the even less demanding diets recommended to the general public by the American Heart Association and other authorities to cut the risk of heart disease: 30 percent of calories from fat and no more than 300 milligrams of cholesterol a day.

Most people can approximate all these diets by: (1) cutting back on servings of red meat, egg yolks, ice cream, cheese (except the low-fat kind) and whole milk; (2) making fruits and nuts the main ingredients of desserts; and (3) increasing intake of vegetables, whole grain foods, fruits, and legumes.

Japanese scientists have also announced that with drugs and diet they were able to stop or reverse artery damage in 167 people. Reportedly, the diet contained very little fat and cholesterol—no animal fats, no cheeses, no butter, very little milk, and no more than one egg daily.

In the Netherlands, investigators report that during a two-year period, artery lesions in 18 people under treatment either remained unchanged or got smaller. The treatment: a vegetarian diet containing twice as much polyunsaturated fat as saturated fat and no more than 100 milligrams of cholesterol per day.

The Dietary Wild Cards

If these studies are any indication, a regression diet must contain far less fat and cholesterol than many people are used to. But if the aim is to reduce blood cholesterol enough to reverse artery damage, there may be ways to make such diets effective *and* easy to live with. Scientists are now investigating two nutritional factors that may lower blood cholesterol much better than anybody expected.

Water-soluble fiber. A growing stack of research suggests that water-soluble dietary fiber—the kind abundant in oats, fruits, barley, and beans—can dramatically affect cholesterol in your blood. It can lower total and LDL cholesterol (an extremely harmful kind) and raise HDL cholesterol (a beneficial type).

Right now, scientists are particularly interested in a water-soluble fiber called guar gum, an additive in many foods.

"In studies we've conducted," says John Farquhar, M.D., director of Stanford University's Center for Research in Disease Prevention, "guar gum seems to significantly lower cholesterol, and other research institutions have had the same results. In fact, guar gum appears to lower cholesterol more substantially than fish oils or other dietary additives."

Monounsaturates. Scientists have already shown that polyunsaturated fats (predominant in safflower, corn, and other vegetable oils) lower cholesterol. They also assumed that monounsaturated fats (abundant in olive and peanut oil) didn't do much of anything to cholesterol. But now research suggests that monounsaturates may lower cholesterol as well as the polyunsaturates do.

Regardless of whether anyone ever perfects a regression diet, the very fact that reversal of heart disease now seems possible will reverberate through the world for years.

"It's a marvelous instinct to want to have bad things like disease simply melt away," says one researcher. Now, at last, the instinct may come face to face with reality.

CHAPTER 5

21st-Century Medical Tests You May Need Now

The American College of Radiology explains ten diagnostic procedures—what they are and how they work.

True or false? (1) Some tests done by radiologists don't involve radiation and are completely harmless. (2) One of the latest developments in radiology is a huge doughnut-shaped magnet. (3) You may take a bigger health risk by avoiding an x-ray exam than by having one. (4) Computers can transform sound waves into pictures.

The statements are all true. Welcome to modern radiology! Here's a look at the state of the art from experts at the American College of Radiology, which has about 20,000 members in the United States and Canada and disseminates information to the medical profession and the public about developments within the specialty. For more information, write the American College of Radiology, 1891 Preston White Drive, Reston, VA 22091. Or call (703) 648-8900 during regular business hours.

Mammography

The advantage of mammography is that it can detect breast cancer about two years before it's noticeable to the touch. The best and most commonly used method is screen/film mammography. It creates an image on film by way of a screen that emits light in response to x-rays. The good news is that today's x-ray film is much more sensitive than it used to be. That means better pictures at a fraction of the

radiation dose. So don't be screening-shy. Early detection ensures a better prognosis!

The American College of Radiology (ACR) recommends that by age 35 to 40, every woman should have a "baseline" mammogram to provide a profile of her normal breasts for comparison with future examinations. Then, they say, mammograms should be repeated every two years until age 50 and annually after that. The ACR and the American Cancer Society urge women to request mammograms for themselves if they meet these age guidelines. (Monthly self-exam and regular exams by a doctor are also vital in detection of breast cancer.)

Estimated cost: $25 to $200. Radiation dose: about 2 rads for a full mammography consisting of two views of both breasts.

Nuclear Scans

Two types are bone scans and something called ventilation-perfusion scintigraphy (or V-P scanning), which is used to examine the lungs. These tests use radioactive compounds (also called radioisotopes or radionuclides), which attach to certain body tissues. After a radioisotope is introduced into the body, the person is positioned under a large instrument called a gamma camera. This device maps the distribution of the radioisotope in the body by translating it into spots of light that expose film.

Radiologists use bone scans to check the skeleton for tumors, infections, injury, or unexplained pain. The scan will point up "hot spots"—areas of increased activity that indicate abnormalities in bony structures—weeks to months before they can be detected by standard x-rays.

Although a bone scan is extremely sensitive, it is far less specific than an x-ray, says Lawrence R. Muroff, M.D., director of nuclear medicine, computerized axial tomography, and magnetic resonance imaging at the University Community Hospital and a clinical professor of radiology at the University of Southern Florida College of Medicine in Tampa. Any hot spot will be followed up with an x-ray. "You're not necessarily saving the patient from getting an x-ray. You're saving the patient from getting lots of unnecessary x-rays," he says. The radioisotope commonly used

in bone scanning is technetium-99m, a material with a half-life of only 6 hours. It leaves the body rapidly, keeping radiation exposure to a minimum.

A similar technique, ventilation-perfusion scintigraphy, can provide physicians with valuable information about the lungs. Ventilation refers to breathing; perfusion is blood flow. Both can be measured using radioisotopes and a gamma camera, says Philip O. Alderson, M.D., professor and vice-chairman of the Department of Radiology and director of the Division of Nuclear Medicine at Columbia-Presbyterian Medical Center in New York City. By comparing the two measurements and looking for a "V-P mismatch," radiologists can detect pulmonary embolism, a potentially fatal condition involving blood clots in the lungs—and beat it to the punch.

Estimated cost: $200 to $300 for bone scan; $400 to $500 for V-P scan. Radiation dose: less than 1 rad for bone scan; about ½ rad to the lungs for V-P scan.

Radioimmunoassay (RIA)

This test can determine the body's level of hormones, vitamins, or a vital drug. Amounts as tiny as one-billionth of a gram can be measured using this safe and ingenious procedure, says Dr. Muroff. Let's say you want to measure the amount of a vitamin in a sample of blood or urine. A biological compound (like an antibody or a protein) that can bind to the vitamin is attached to radioactive molecules. The compound is mixed into the blood or urine and links up with the vitamin. Because the compound is "tagged" with radioactivity, it can be easily found and measured. Bonus: The entire procedure takes place outside the body, involving no radiation exposure whatever!

Estimated cost: $10 to $15. Radiation dose: none.

Digital Subtraction Angiography (DSA)

Angiography has been used for years to help doctors diagnose clogged arteries and head off strokes. After injecting contrast dye into the artery through a catheter, radiologists

can pinpoint potential trouble spots. Now, a recent advance in imaging, called DSA, has become an important complement to angiography.

With this technique, unwanted x-ray detail is subtracted from the image, offering radiologists a clearer outline of the veins and arteries. In addition, DSA requires less contrast material to produce an image. This means that narrower, more comfortable catheters can be used—and, best of all, there's less radiation exposure for you.

Estimated cost: $500 to $1,000. Radiation dose: approximately 1 rad, depending on the area studied.

Computerized Axial Tomography (CAT or CT)

Take an x-ray tube and a fixed ring of very sensitive detectors, add a computer, and you've got the "granddaddy" of modern imaging: the CAT scanner.

Called the biggest imaging advance since the discovery of x-rays, the CAT scanner looks like a giant washing machine. What it does is create detailed two-dimensional pictures of the entire body so that three-dimensional images can be created. After x-rays scan the body, a computer converts these findings into digital form. That information is then turned into an image, which is projected onto a TV screen. The entire process takes just 40 seconds.

The CAT scanner can distinguish tumors from nearby soft tissues, determining their size and volume in the process. The brain and liver can be imaged. Scanning the skull, chest, and abdomen of a trauma victim can provide prompt diagnosis and speed the treatment of any internal injuries, notes Stanley Baum, M.D., professor and chairman of the Department of Radiology at the University of Pennsylvania in Philadelphia.

Estimated cost: $300 to $400. Radiation dose: less than 1 rad.

Magnetic Resonance Imaging (MRI)

Meet the MRI machine—a powerful magnetic coil, up to 30,000 times the strength of the earth's magnetic field.

Unlike a standard x-ray or CAT scan, this machine uses no ionizing radiation, no radioactive material. And, as far as the experts know, it involves no risks or side effects. It performs its magic with an ingenious combination of magnetic field, radio waves, and computer, providing anatomic images in multiple planes.

The subject is placed inside the magnetic coil—a daunting thought, but the procedure is completely painless. Protons (the nuclei of the hydrogen atom) in the body line up in response to the magnet. Then a radio transmitter sends pulses that excite the nuclei, causing them to move out of formation and emit a signal. When the transmitter is shut off, the hydrogen nuclei stand at attention once again. Having "watched" this whole procedure and gathered information throughout the test, the computer now translates its findings into diagnostic images. (Interestingly, the only known risk associated with MRI is accidents in the room, notes Dr. Baum—a stethoscope will be pulled into the machine with the force of a bullet.)

Useful in the study of musculoskeletal diseases, MRI also has the potential to detect changes in joint tissue early on, so that people with rheumatoid arthritis and osteoarthritis can get the jump on treatment. A tumor or large cystic spaces within the spinal cord can be detected. MRI may also be used to study biochemical activity in tissue at the early stages of disease.

Estimated cost: $600 to $800. Radiation dose: none.

Sonography, or Ultrasound

Here's another exciting alternative to ionizing radiation: high-frequency sound waves. The key component is the transducer, a device that converts electrical energy into sound waves. As the transducer is held over the area in question, the waves bounce off structures within the body and echo back to the transducer. This information is then electronically transformed into a picture.

Ultrasound's value lies in its ability to examine soft-tissue densities and discriminate among them. "It's an indicator as to which lesions need to be studied further," says George R. Leopold, M.D., professor and chairman of

radiology at the University of California at San Diego. Suspicious lumps and gallstones can be imaged by a sonogram. It's used in pregnancy because it poses no radiation risk.

Future developments: The use of ultrasound to study not only the structure of blood vessels but also the flow within vessels. A new technique may allow urologists and radiologists to recognize early cancer of the prostate.

Estimated cost: $100 to $300. Radiation dose: none.

Doppler Flow Imaging (Duplex Doppler)

If you've ever listened to the declining pitch of a train's whistle as the train disappears down the track, you've observed the Doppler effect: The pitch of a sound rises as the source approaches and decreases as it moves away. Recently, the same principle has been applied to the study of blood flow, resulting in the creation of a Doppler ultrasound beam. "If the beam hits a moving target, the signal we get back is altered," explains Dr. Leopold. Instead of a picture, the Doppler beam produces a tracing of peaks and valleys. Linked with ultrasound images, it is used to evaluate blood flow, even in deep vessels of the body.

Color Doppler flow imaging, the latest development in Doppler testing, samples all areas of flow within the vessel simultaneously. By assigning a different color to each flow speed, the radiologist can quickly spot areas of slowdown or blockage.

Estimated cost: $200. Radiation dose: none.

Single Photon Emission Computed Tomography (SPECT)

When coronary artery disease is suspected, testing with the help of SPECT can be particularly useful in evaluating the condition of the heart muscle. A remarkable imaging technique, SPECT features three innovations: Its gamma camera rotates to shoot from a variety of angles, it produces images of thin sections of the body, and the computer produces a three-dimensional picture.

To prepare for this test, the subject exercises to get the heart in gear. (An EKG helps monitor the activity.) Then a radioactive tracer, such as thallium-201, is introduced into the body. "The heart is a big muscle surrounded by a lot of air," says Dr. Alderson. "When you inject thallium, it's

Minimizing Your Radiation Risks

The risk you take with a test involving radiation depends on many factors, including the techniques and equipment used, the area of the body exposed (the thyroid is more sensitive to radiation than muscle or skin, for example), and the kind of x-ray exam involved (a gastrointestinal, or GI, series exposes you to much more radiation than do dental x-rays).

To minimize the risks:

- Make sure that the test is necessary. Ask your doctor whether his or her treatment plan will change depending on the results of the test. If it won't, the test may not be necessary.
- Make sure the testing facility is under the supervision of a full-time, board-certified radiologist.
- If you're having a mammogram, ask if the facility uses "dedicated" equipment (that is, equipment designed exclusively for breast exams) and if the equipment is calibrated regularly. It should be calibrated at least once, and preferably twice, a year.
- Avoid exposure to old-fashioned fluoroscopes.
- Finally, consider the big picture. Is this test worth the risk you may be taking? Routine chest x-rays, for example, are now widely regarded as unnecessary.

On the other hand, overcautiousness about radiation risk could keep you away from a test that might detect a serious medical problem and save your life.

pretty easy to see the heart muscle." Pictures are taken with the SPECT machine, the subject waits several hours, and more pictures are taken. Together, the two sets of images indicate any blockage in the heart that may be causing angina or other troublesome symptoms.

Estimated cost: $600 to $800. Radiation dose: less than 1 rad.

Positron Emission Tomography (PET)

Beyond the imaging of anatomy, soft tissues, and blood flow enters a technique that uses radioactive tracers to take a look at the metabolic activity going on inside an organ.

The brain and the heart have been prime targets for this promising new test, according to David E. Kuhl, M.D., professor of internal medicine and radiology and chief of the Division of Nuclear Medicine at the University of Michigan Hospital in Ann Arbor, and Markus Schwaiger, M.D., associate professor of internal medicine in the Divisions of Nuclear Medicine and Cardiology at the University of Michigan Hospital. Radiologists can use PET to study brain-related disorders such as epilepsy, Alzheimer's disease, schizophrenia, and Parkinson's disease. The vitality of the heart tissue can also be evaluated—an important test before surgery.

Estimated cost: not yet available (PET is still considered experimental). Radiation dose: to evaluate vitality of heart tissue, whole-body exposure is about ½ rad.

What's a Rad?

A rad is a unit of measurement that describes the dose of radiation absorbed by an exposed object or body. Sometimes doctors use another measurement called a rem, which is roughly equivalent to a rad. Mammograms and x-rays aren't the only sources of radiation, however. The average American receives 0.36 rad a year, over half of which comes from natural sources.

CHAPTER 6
Get Rid of Hemorrhoids—for Good

Don't just put up with discomfort or pain. You and your doctor can now choose from a half dozen safe procedures.

"And they had emerods [hemorrhoids] in their secret parts . . . and the cry . . . went up to heaven."

That comes from the Bible (1 Samuel 5:9–12), so rest assured that hemorrhoids have been raising cain for quite some time. There's even a patron saint for hemorrhoid sufferers—St. Fiacre.

Spiritual relief aside, however, modern medicine has been making impressive inroads against the age-old agony of hemorrhoids (also called piles, from the Latin word *pila,* meaning "ball"). First, however, a quick look at what causes the hellish swellings.

Although heredity, heavy lifting, prolonged periods of sitting or standing, and hypertension within the liver also can contribute to the dreaded affliction, the most common cause of hemorrhoids is simple constipation—straining at something that Mother Nature didn't *intend* to be an eye-bulging experience.

"Exercise is great, but not on the john," says bowel specialist Lester Rosen, M.D., from Allentown, Pennsylvania. Delicate tissue inside or outside the anus gets overengorged with blood, and blood vessels can rupture, causing further swelling. Result: You've got yourself a hemorrhoid (an internal one if the swelling occurs inside the anus or an external one if it occurs outside).

Fiber to the Rescue

And the most common cause of hemorrhoid-producing constipation? A shortage of roughage (fiber) in the diet. "There's no question that more fiber in most people's diets could substantially reduce their hemorrhoidal risks," Dr. Rosen says. "Fiber also is important for helping to speed recovery for existing cases of hemorrhoids. It does this primarily by making stools softer, more voluminous, and easier to pass." (See the table "Foods That Can Fight Hemorrhoids" on page 52 for the best fiber sources.)

Something in the neighborhood of 20 to 25 grams of fiber a day is what most experts recommend, not just for a happier bottom but for weight control and a healthier heart as well. Getting more liquids into the diet (alcohol not included) also can help make stools softer and less challenging to pass, Dr. Rosen says.

Go or Get Off the Pot

Yet another correctable contributor to hemorrhoids can be using the toilet for other than strictly bowel-related business. "I tell my patients not to make their bathrooms their libraries," Dr. Rosen says.

It seems that just the act of sitting on a toilet can put undue pressure on the blood vessels of the anal area—yet another reason not to be constipated.

"People should try to restrict their toilet time to a maximum of 5 minutes," Dr. Rosen advises. "You've either got a problem or you're risking one if you sit for much longer than that." And he recommends clearing your toilet area of all literature as a way of encouraging speedier bathroom experiences.

Visit Your Doc, Not Your Drugstore

And what about one of those highly touted (on TV) salves for alleviating hemorrhoidal woes?

The promises made by those ads have us spending an estimated $200 million annually on over-the-counter hem-

Foods That Can Fight Hemorrhoids

Most people could reduce their hemorrhoid risk by increasing the amount of fiber in their diets. Twenty to 25 grams of dietary fiber a day is what most experts recommend. The following foods are your best fiber sources.

Food (3½ oz.)	**Fiber** (g.)	**Food** (3½ oz.)	**Fiber** (g.)
Beans		*Fruits*	
Kidney beans, cooked	7.9	Figs	16.9
Baked beans, with tomato sauce	7.3	Prunes	11.9
Navy beans, cooked	6.3	Raisins	8.7
Lima beans, canned	5.4	Apricots, dried	8.1
Peas, dried, cooked	4.7	Dates	7.6
Lentils, cooked	3.7	Raspberries	5.1
		Pears, with skin	2.8
		Blueberries	2.7
		Apples, with skin	2.5
		Peaches, with skin	2.1
		Oranges	2.0
Breads and Pasta			
Rye crispbread	14.9	*Nuts*	
Wheat crispbread	12.9	Peanuts	8.1
Bran muffins	6.3	Almonds	7.2
Whole wheat bread	5.7	Filberts	6.0
Cracked wheat bread	4.1		
Mixed grain bread	3.7	*Vegetables*	
Pumpernickel bread	3.2	Peas	4.5
Oatmeal	2.2	Parsnips	3.5
		Brussels sprouts	3.0
		Carrots	3.0
Flours and Grains		Broccoli	2.8
Corn bran	62.2	Corn, canned	2.8
Wheat bran	41.2	Green beans	2.6
Oat bran	27.8		
Rye flour	12.8		
Whole wheat flour	8.9		

orrhoid medications, but most doctors agree that their abilities are highly exaggerated. Those intended merely to keep the anal area clean (such as Tucks and Balneol pads) may be worthwhile, Dr. Rosen says, but products designed to "shrink hemorrhoidal tissue" or "relieve the pain and itching" are of limited or temporary value.

"Perhaps the biggest danger with these products is that they can keep people from seeing their doctors for conditions that could be more serious than hemorrhoids," Dr. Rosen says. "Rectal bleeding can be a sign of colorectal cancer, for example, a cancer that is highly curable—but only if diagnosed in time."

So by all means, if you see blood in your toilet, see your doctor. Chances are that hemorrhoids are all that's involved and that you will be advised of the following treatments.

Relief for "Minor" Cases

No case feels minor to the person who has it, but doctors do have a classification system for hemorrhoids that designates some as less serious than others. Here's what you're liable to be offered for less than dire (first- or second-degree) cases.

The sitz bath. As old as the hills but effective nonetheless, the sitz bath—which involves simply sitting in 3 or 4 inches of warm (not hot) water in a bathtub—is especially suited for external hemorrhoids. Several tablespoons of Epsom salts can make the sitz bath even more soothing.

Witch hazel. This remedy is also for external hemorrhoids and is "as effective as any highly advertised TV remedy for relieving pain and itching," according to Dr. Rosen.

Sclerotherapy. Indicated for first-degree and small second-degree internal hemorrhoids, sclerotherapy has been more popular in England than the United States but has met with success nonetheless. Hemorrhoids are injected with a 5 percent solution of phenol in almond oil and wither away as a result.

Help for More Serious Cases

If your doctor determines that your hemorrhoid problem is

more severe, it may be necessary to consider one of the following treatments.

Rubber-band ligation. Probably the most widely used office procedure, ligation (or banding) is suitable for internal hemorrhoids of the first, second, and third degrees. Hemorrhoids are tied at their upper end with an elastic band, usually not more than a few at a time, with a three-week interval between bandings. Within 7 to 20 days, the strangled hemorrhoids "die" and fall off, usually with a minimum of pain and bleeding. Risks of bleeding and infection exist, but they are small. The procedure should *not* be used on people taking anticoagulants (blood-thinning medications) or people with compromised immune status or portal hypertension.

Infrared photocoagulation. Also an office procedure, this involves zapping hemorrhoids with infrared heat, which causes blood within the hemorrhoid to coagulate and the hemorrhoid itself to collapse. Allegedly less painful than banding, the procedure may not be as effective or free of complications as ligation.

Cryotherapy. Not as popular as it was during the 1960s, cryotherapy involves the destruction of both internal and external hemorrhoids by freezing. Because results seem to vary widely with the experience of the doctor wielding the freeze-wand, the method has gradually fallen out of favor and currently is thought to be less advisable than surgery.

Laser therapy. Controversy continues to surround the effectiveness of this technique, which shoots internal hemorrhoids with bolts of electromagnetic radiation directed through a flexible tube. Conservative practitioners say the technique has yet to prove itself any better than surgery, though the therapy is widely promoted and practiced by its proponents.

Electric current. This method of hemorrhoid execution involves shocking the internal hemorrhoidal base with low-power DC current delivered by a probe. First-degree hemorrhoids require about a 6-minute shock, while fourth-degree ones require about 9 minutes per treatment (two or three are usually needed). The electrocuted tissue dies and detaches itself in 3 to 10 days, no scarring occurs, and the procedure requires only a topical anesthetic. In one

study of 42 patients, the procedure proved 100 percent successful in all cases.

Surgery. And last but certainly not least, the knife. "It's an unfounded myth that surgery for hemorrhoids is a great disaster," Dr. Rosen says. "My patients receive a local anesthetic and usually can leave the hospital, pain-free, the next day."

CHAPTER 7

Best Remedies for Six Beastly Headaches

Identify the kind that pain you, then relieve them with the right treatment.

Not long ago, if you had an aching head and your doctor couldn't find a cause, he might send you to the psychiatrist across the hall. Luckily, those days are over. Headache diagnosis and treatment have become a medical specialty. Doctors are discovering more kinds of headaches all the time and learning how to treat them. That makes it easier than ever to find relief for *your* special headache.

Here's what leading experts have to say about some not-so-common kinds of headaches.

The Sinus Headache

A real sinus headache is a gnawing pain, swelling, or tenderness over the forehead, nose, or cheek. It's caused by an acute infection of the sinuses, ears, or teeth and is usually accompanied by fever and nasal discharge.

Such headaches are rare. Migraine and cluster headaches (which cause severe pain and occur in groups) are often misdiagnosed as sinus headaches.

"Most people who get aching pain around their sinuses do not actually have a sinus headache. They have what we call 'vasomotor rhinitis,' " says Seymour Diamond, M.D., director of the country's oldest and largest private headache clinic, the Diamond Headache Clinic, in Chicago. "The blood vessels in the area around their nose and sinuses are somehow stimulated to constrict or swell, setting off pain." Air pollution, changes in the weather, or certain allergies can cause this reaction.

Many people with vasomotor rhinitis find over-the-counter decongestants helpful, because these drugs constrict blood vessels. And their occasional use is fine. But prolonged or frequent use can lead to dependency on those medications.

"A decongestant may help your headache. But unless you have the symptoms of a true sinus headache, like fever and discharge, you should be taking aspirin, acetaminophen, or ibuprofen—but not on a daily basis—for these headaches," Dr. Diamond says.

If you really do have a sinus headache with fever and discharge, see your doctor. Antibiotics, decongestants, and possibly anti-inflammatory drugs will be prescribed to drain and heal your sinuses. Putting a hot, wet towel over your face or inhaling steam may help, too. Sometimes surgical drainage is needed.

The Allergy Headache

Is your pain accompanied by a stuffy nose and watery eyes? You may have an inhalant allergy headache. But if food sensitivities are causing your symptoms, your headache is more likely to resemble a common migraine, with throbbing pain, dizziness, and sensitivity to light and noise. In fact, some people with migraines say certain foods trigger their symptoms.

Antihistamines or allergy shots may relieve inhalant allergy headaches. For food sensitivities, being a good detective is your best bet. Red wine or other alcohol, aged

cheeses, hot baked goods (made with yeast), monosodium glutamate (MSG), caffeine, and nitrites (in lunch meats and hot dogs) are among the most commonly accused headache-producing foods.

Sexual Headaches

Yes, you read correctly. For some people, passion and pain are cruelly linked. In most, the headache begins around the moment of orgasm, with a sudden throbbing similar to that of a migraine. In others, the pain starts a few minutes before orgasm, intensifying as climax nears. The pain resembles the dull ache of a muscle-tension headache.

"These headaches are very frightening, of course, and most doctors would do a brain scan, and maybe even an angiogram, to make sure the patient doesn't have a brain aneurysm [dangerously weakened blood vessels]," says Robert S. Kunkel, Jr., M.D., director of the Cleveland Clinic's Headache Center. "It's very important to have this checked out, even though in most cases it won't be that."

The truth is, doctors don't really know what causes sexual headaches. "Most of us feel it's some sort of vascular type of headache, caused by a sudden increase in blood pressure at the time of orgasm," Dr. Kunkel says. "Or it could be related to hormone changes or muscle tension."

For people who have these headaches regularly, doctors may prescribe beta-blockers, drugs that reduce blood pressure. Taking ergotamine, a drug that prevents blood vessel dilation, shortly before having sex is also sometimes recommended. And anti-inflammatory drugs, such as Indocin or Motrin, have been reported to be helpful in people who have these headaches almost every time they have sex.

"Reassurance and relaxation therapy can also work wonders," Dr. Kunkel says.

The Glare or Eyestrain Headache

Pain from eyestrain headaches occurs in the face around the eyes and affects both sides equally. Since it can also be caused by glaucoma, it's wise to have the pressure in your eyeballs checked if you begin to have this kind of pain, Dr.

Diamond says. Glaucoma can cause permanent damage to the eye.

When you squint or use your eyes too much, the eye muscles go into a state of contraction and begin to ache. That is what causes the headache. Give your eyes a break. Have your vision checked to see if you need stronger glasses. If glare is your problem, wear sunglasses or a hat with a visor so that you can avoid squinting.

The Hunger Headache

"I call this 'the weekend headache,' " Dr. Diamond says. This is pain caused by strenuous dieting, skipping a meal, or, as Dr. Diamond suggests, by sleeping so late you postpone breakfast until the early hours of the afternoon.

Low blood sugar or other body changes associated with hunger trigger this headache, and the treatment is simple, Dr. Diamond says: Develop a set pattern of living habits. "We tell people with these headaches to get up at the same time, even on weekends. They should eat something, go to the bathroom, and then go back to bed if they want."

Some "hunger" headaches are actually the result of caffeine withdrawal. In that case, a cup of coffee or a cola may help your headache.

The Menstrual Headache

If a woman is prone to getting headaches, especially migraines, she's most likely to get them immediately before or during her menstrual period. These headaches are caused by hormone changes.

"If over-the-counter painkillers work, then that's fine," Dr. Kunkel says. For more severe cases, he will prescribe a nonsteroidal anti-inflammatory drug, to be taken only during the time the headaches are most likely to occur. Some doctors also prescribe a hormone, progesterone, in extreme cases.

Finally, doctors agree that almost any kind of headache will feel better if you can relax. Try rolling your head slowly from side to side. Shrug, then drop your shoulders. Take deep, long, calming breaths. Imagine the pain leaving

your head as you exhale. Or go for a brisk walk to literally "clear your head." Aerobic exercise increases the oxygen flow to your brain and can help relieve even a stubborn headache for some people.

CHAPTER 8
Q & A: Ten Tough Ones!

Experts answer the questions that worry you about AIDS, aspirin, Alzheimer's, and more.

Q. *I've been married for 20 years. I am monogamous. Am I totally protected against AIDS, or is there something I've overlooked that could put me at risk for exposure to the virus?*

A. Assuming neither of you is an intravenous drug user, only two circumstances might put you at risk for AIDS. First, although you have been faithful, did your spouse commit any infidelities—either heterosexual or homosexual—over the past seven to ten years? If so, there's the slight chance of contact with a carrier. The Centers for Disease Control in Atlanta have documented new cases of AIDS as many as seven years after exposure.

Blood transfusions pose the second risk. A screening process for blood donors has been in effect since 1985, but it's not a catchall. AIDS antibodies can take anywhere from two weeks to several months to form. So a recently infected donor may be tested as "safe" today, but the virus could develop in the blood later. About 2 percent of patients with AIDS got it through a transfusion. A precaution: Store your own blood in advance if you know you'll be having elective surgery.

Q. *There is a definite history of osteoporosis in my family, so I want to do everything I can to prevent it. I exercise and get the RDA of calcium. Should I also be taking estrogen?*

A. "Estrogen excels as a preventive measure for osteoporosis," says Robert Lindsay, M.D., Ph.D., director of research at New York's Helen Hayes Hospital and one of the country's leading osteoporosis investigators. "It can't build new bone to replace what has already been lost, but it can stop any further bone loss." Estrogen can reduce the risk of hip fractures by as much as half, and may even protect against cardiovascular disease.

If you've reached menopause, now is the best time to consider estrogen therapy to make up for what your ovaries aren't contributing anymore. You should discuss the benefits versus the possible risks of estrogen therapy with your doctor.

Q. *I've read I should cut back on sun exposure. But won't I be risking vitamin D deficiency by avoiding those rays?*

A. It takes only a few minutes of summer sun on your face and hands to bestow plenty of this nutrient. If you *always* use a strong sunscreen or block, however, you might possibly be robbing your bones of vitamin D. Researchers at Southern Illinois University School of Medicine recently found that using a PABA sunscreen with a sun protection factor of 8 dramatically reduced the skin's ability to produce vitamin D. They suggest you get regular unscreened doses of low-level sunlight, from early morning or late afternoon rays. That way, you'll be balancing the sun's harmful and beneficial effects. Getting enough vitamin D from weak winter sunlight can be difficult, however, so it might be smart to drink more fortified milk or to take a supplement during those months.

Q. *My 56-year-old uncle is showing early signs of Alzheimer's disease—confusion and memory loss. What are the prospects for a meaningful breakthrough in the treatment of Alzheimer's in the next five years?*

A. "We're not likely to see a definitive treatment that will either prevent or reverse the memory and thinking disorders of Alzheimer's disease within the next 5 years,

and probably not for the next 10 to 20 years," says David Drachman, M.D., chairman of the Department of Neurology at the University of Massachusetts Medical School.

Scientists are a long way from understanding Alzheimer's disease. And before definitive treatment can begin, researchers must first find what causes it. "Possible causes now under investigation," says Dr. Drachman, "include genetic disorders, viruses, toxic substances, and factors that alter or accelerate the aging process of the brain."

Besides research efforts to understand and treat the disease, a Congressional advisory committee, of which Dr. Drachman is a member, has just been established to examine strategies for coping with the care and expense of Alzheimer's patients.

For more information on the disease, contact Alzheimer's Disease and Related Disorders Association, Inc., 70 East Lake Street, Suite 600, Chicago, IL 60601 or call 1-800-621-0379 outside Illinois or 1-800-572-6037 in Illinois.

Q. *What can I do to prevent cataracts from developing? There's a history of them in my family.*

A. Start by wearing sunglasses when you're skiing, gardening, walking—anytime you're in the sun. They'll help protect you from the harmful rays suspected of playing a role in later cataract formation. Look for sunglasses that block a high percentage of ultraviolet light.

In research labs, vitamin C is showing promise against cataracts. One study under way now is investigating the possible anticataract effect of vitamin C in humans. (Research has previously been with guinea pigs.) And three population studies either under way or about to be published suggest diets with enhanced levels of carotenes and vitamin C may delay the onset of some cataracts by acting as antioxidants. Antioxidants appear to counteract the damaging effect of light and oxygen.

Q. *I was always thin. Then I had three children. The last was born five years ago, but I still weigh 35 pounds more than I should. Does pregnancy change your metabolism?*

A. You did have excess hormones in your body while

you were pregnant that conspired against your figure. They encouraged fat cells to form and be stored. But once each of your babies was born, the hormones subsided and bowed out of any blame for your excess weight.

So what's the problem? Chances are you're not as active as you were before your pregnancies. "Although you may feel as though you've never been *more* active in your life since you have children to care for, you may not be getting the right kinds of exercise—the kinds that keep your metabolic rate humming along," says Mona Shangold, M.D., director of the sports gynecology center at Georgetown University.

Aerobic exercise (such as swimming or walking) and strength training (such as weight lifting) build muscle mass. "Muscle tissue has a faster metabolic rate than fat tissue; this means it burns more calories," explains Dr. Shangold, who is also coauthor of *The Complete Sports Medicine Book for Women.* "So a 120-pound woman who is fat will burn fewer calories than a 120-pound woman who is muscular." If you are exercising aerobically and still can't seem to lose weight, you may want to have your doctor check for other problems that may have developed *unrelated* to your pregnancies.

Q. *I'm confused. I've read iron is important to maintain a healthy body, but I've also read that iron has been shown to impair the immune system. What am I supposed to do?*

A. Just be sure to continue getting the Recommended Dietary Allowance of iron each day. (That's 10 milligrams for men, 18 for women up to age 50, and 10 for women 50 and older.)

It's true that an excess of iron can leave you more vulnerable to infectious bacteria. But the reason has more to do with the fact that too much iron helps bacteria to multiply, rather than directly damaging your immune system. Iron deficiency, on the other hand, *won't* keep you healthier by "starving out" bacteria. It will only keep the various components of your immune system operating half-heartedly because they'll be experiencing a shortage of oxygen. Delivering oxygen is iron's main job.

Q. *I can't possibly take the time to do all the things recommended by doctors these days. Of the following, which three health steps should I focus on?*

- *Exercising regularly.*
- *Eating a high-fiber diet.*
- *Reducing dietary fat and cholesterol.*
- *Taking vitamins.*
- *Lowering sodium intake.*
- *Cutting down on stress.*
- *Increasing calcium intake.*
- *Limiting alcohol consumption.*
- *Eating more fish.*
- *Eating more foods rich in beta-carotene.*

A. All of these steps are important. But if you're going to start the journey to better health by first mastering three, try these multibenefit measures. (Later, when they become an integral part of your life, you can tackle the others.)

Exercise regularly. Some of the benefits: You'll lose weight by burning calories and raising your metabolic rate. Losing weight will help lower your blood pressure, and it will help reduce artery-clogging LDL cholesterol while boosting beneficial HDL cholesterol. That lowers your risk of heart disease. Your cardiovascular system will become stronger, giving you a faster recovery time after exercise (in other words, it'll get easier), and a lower resting heart rate (meaning your heart won't have to work as hard to pump blood when you're not exercising). Finally, exercise is thought to help ward off osteoporosis, and it can also reduce excess stress.

Eat more fiber. The American Cancer Society strongly recommends this step to guard against the risk of colon cancer. One reason: Fiber is thought to shorten the travel time of waste through the bowel, so that carcinogens (cancer-causing agents) are moved out before they can cause trouble. If you eat more fiber-rich foods, such as grains, vegetables, and fruit, you should automatically eat less fat. So you're likely to lose weight. And eating less fat means you'll lower your cholesterol intake as well.

Reduce dietary fat and cholesterol. A good move, considering that about half the people in this country die of

cardiovascular disease. If you follow the experts' advice to reduce the amount of fat in your diet to about 30 percent of calories (instead of the 40 percent most people are getting now), you'll probably get your cholesterol down to acceptable levels. And since you'll be choosing substitute foods from healthier, lower-calorie food groups, such as the ones mentioned earlier, you should lose weight at the same time.

Q. *Is moderate alcohol consumption good or bad?*

A. The idea that moderate drinking promotes health had been based on a few intriguing studies that indicated alcohol raises heart-protecting HDL cholesterol. But a recent British study of almost 8,000 men found that although alcohol does indeed raise HDL levels, it seems to be quite unimportant in affecting risk of heart disease one way or the other. Risk factors like smoking and high blood pressure were judged far more relevant than drinking.

What's more, as several experts concluded in the *Journal of the American Medical Association,* "Even if moderate drinking were shown conclusively to reduce the risk of heart disease, recommendations to increase alcohol consumption . . . would be ill-advised because of overriding considerations regarding other health concerns."

The risk posed by alcohol for breast cancer, for example, is sobering. Two recent studies involving more than 97,000 women found those who drank even moderate amounts of alcohol had a greater risk of breast cancer than women who didn't drink. And the risk for hemorrhagic stroke more than doubles even for "light" drinkers, who average less than one drink per day.

In addition, moderate amounts of alcohol can trigger reactions in people taking sedatives, tranquilizers, painkillers, and over-the-counter medications. All in all, it's not a picture to raise your spirits.

Q. *Should I take aspirin for my heart or not, and what's the right dose?*

A. Only your doctor can answer this for you. If you have patterns of heart pain called unstable angina, doctors believe you can help control the condition and reduce your

risk of heart attack by taking one adult-strength aspirin tablet (325 milligrams) every other day.

This same dose may also help you avoid a second heart attack if one has already occurred. Likewise, if you have what doctors call cerebrovascular insufficiency, or ministrokes, you may benefit from aspirin. Again, consult your physician.

However, if you're clear of any signs of coronary artery disease, there's no conclusive evidence you'll protect yourself by starting aspirin therapy now. A lot of researchers think there *might* be a preventive advantage, though, and are conducting studies to find out. One study currently under way involves over 20,000 healthy physicians who have volunteered to take either aspirin or a lookalike placebo every other day for several years.

PART III: HEALTH-SAVING ADVANCES

CHAPTER 9

The Stroke-Stopping Power of Potassium

Fruits and vegetables may stack the odds against this major killer.

Stroke is the tornado of cardiovascular diseases—feared by many, it hits quickly and unexpectedly, leaving survivors and their families in upheaval.

The third leading cause of death in the United States, stroke often entails a slow fight to regain speech and movement capabilities for those who do survive. Nearly two-thirds may be handicapped afterward. This is one reason why many stroke patients never return to work.

As serious as stroke is, however, a simple, sensible step is showing promise as a protector against it. Evidence shows you may have a better chance of avoiding stroke by getting more of the nutrient potassium in your diet. Studies have suggested people with a higher intake of fruits and vegetables rich in potassium may actually have a reduced risk of stroke-associated death.

Imagine you're giving someone mouth-to-mouth resuscitation—that person is dependent on you until medical help arrives. If you stop, he may die. Your brain has this

same dependent partnership with your heart. Twenty-five percent of the blood pumped by your heart is sent via arteries to your brain, which needs an uninterrupted supply to function. If this blood flow is diminished from either a clot blocking an artery or a ruptured blood vessel, your brain cells lose their source of energy and begin to die. This is the heart of a stroke.

Until recently, high blood pressure was just about the only thing the medical community could pinpoint as being a major risk factor for stroke. Doctors put hypertensive patients on pressure-taming medication as a preventive step.

Recent studies, however, show a different picture.

A 12-year study of diet and stroke incidence among 850 Californians was conducted jointly by researchers from the University of California at San Diego (UCSD) School of Medicine and the University of Cambridge School of Medicine in England.

After more than a decade of following the subjects, the doctors found a startling correlation between one factor and the incidence of stroke-related deaths. It *wasn't* just blood pressure.

"The people who had strokes did have the well-documented excess of high blood pressure," says Elizabeth Barrett-Connor, M.D., chairman of the Department of Community and Family Medicine at the UCSD School of Medicine. "But the total picture went above and beyond the association with hypertension."

Potassium was the key.

The diets the subjects had reported were divided into three categories—low, average, and high intakes of potassium. At the study's end, people who consumed the least had the highest number of stroke-associated deaths in that 12-year period. But not one stroke-associated death occurred in the people whose diets contained the highest levels of potassium.

About a 400-milligram increase in potassium intake was associated with a 40 percent reduction in the risk of stroke-associated mortality. "That's roughly the amount in one additional daily serving of a potassium-rich fruit or vegetable," explains Dr. Barrett-Connor.

Call in the "K"

"There is evidence that the elevated blood pressure probably isn't so much the cause of stroke as it is a symptom of some other stroke-provoking condition," explains Richard D. Moore, M.D., Ph.D., professor of biophysics at the State University of New York and visiting professor of physiology and biophysics at the University of Vermont School of Medicine. "If high blood pressure were the only factor involved, then people who get their pressure levels down with antihypertensive drugs shouldn't be having any strokes—and they are."

To understand why, we need to consider the role of potassium inside cells. "We're looking at a mineral imbalance in the cells, primarily involving potassium and sodium," says Dr. Moore, who is coauthor of *The K Factor.* The book contends that optimal dietary intake of potassium (K is scientific shorthand for this element) can reverse and prevent high blood pressure.

"It's well known that we need to cut our sodium intake. But a more crucial step is increasing dietary potassium so as to keep these two minerals in the right ratio," Dr. Moore notes. An unbalanced ratio of potassium and sodium can do several things. One involves the small arteries that contract and dilate to regulate your blood pressure.

Sodium and potassium atoms each have an electrical charge attached to them. If there's too much sodium and not enough potassium in the cells surrounding those arteries, an electrical imbalance is created. "This can cause the arteries to clamp down way too hard when they contract. The result can be higher blood pressure, which can strain artery walls, and possibly a slowing of blood flow in some of the small arteries," Dr. Moore says.

This slowed blood flow might make it more possible for a clot to form, he adds. Clots in arteries providing blood to the brain account for two out of every three strokes.

Another function of potassium is regulating the amount of pressure-boosting sodium in cells. Some sodium is necessary for cells to function. But what you take in tends to pool inside cells. A high concentration of pooled sodium increases the chances of your blood pressure rising and

your cell walls weakening. High potassium levels, though, can kick into gear a pumping action that keeps sodium moving out of the cells.

Diet Defense

Based on this evidence, the call is out for us to consume more potassium-rich foods.

Fruits and vegetables are great sources of this nutrient. In addition to their role as stroke defenders, fruits and vegetables also appear to offer significant protection against cardiovascular mortality in general when a greater amount is consumed, according to a 14-year study by University of Mississippi researchers *(Medical Hypotheses).*

"When you combine the findings of our [12-year stroke and diet] study with other scientific findings that point to fruits and vegetables for prevention of cancer and other conditions," explains Dr. Barrett-Connor, "plus the fact that it's a safe step, it's valid to recommend eating more fruits and vegetables rather than taking potassium pills."

"You can also keep sodium intake down and get your potassium levels up by paying attention to the things that throw off your ratio in the first place," says George D. Webb, Ph.D., coauthor with Dr. Moore of *The K Factor* and associate professor of physiology and biophysics at the University of Vermont School of Medicine.

"Three modern food-preparation habits undermine this mineral balance," he notes. "First, there's no need to use salt as a condiment. Second, boiling foods pilfers potassium. Up to 30 percent or more of potassium dissolves out of vegetables this way," Dr. Webb adds. "Often, the canned vegetables we rely on are boiled during processing—and then we boil them again on our stoves." He advises steaming, baking, microwaving, or stir-frying vegetables to retain more potassium.

A third factor creating high sodium levels and low potassium levels is our choice of foods. "We tend to get a high percentage of calories from foods with lots of sugar and lots of fat but little potassium," he says. "Eating vegetables, grains, lean meats, and fruits will help restore the balance you need."

If high blood pressure and stroke are of concern to you, you might look to your diet as a simple line of defense. "It's an easy step," says Dr. Webb, "against serious problems."

CHAPTER 10

Your New Guide to a Healthier Heart

Five Harvard experts offer a new perspective and practical advice.

So maybe you have heard it all before. Maybe you've heard the rules for preventing heart disease so many times you can recite them as easily as the Pledge of Allegiance.

1. Cholesterol's bad, but there's worse to be had.
2. You can walk (or run) and your heart work is done.
3. Salt's not always at fault.

What? Those aren't the rules you remember? Not even close? Don't worry. It's only natural, because our understanding of heart disease, and how to prevent and treat it, is constantly changing and evolving. New research emerges and shades what we know, or displaces it completely.

That's why it's high time for an update. It's time to put a finger on the pulse of heart disease research and report on the very latest findings, opinions, and recommendations.

To get that information, the renowned doctors at Harvard Medical School were consulted. Researchers and clinicians there were interviewed to get their perspective and their recommendations on what's now considered best for your ticker.

A Walk's as Good as a Run

People once thought that any exercise that didn't have you pounding the pavement wouldn't help your heart. If you weren't running or jogging, you were going nowhere. No more. Now we know that simply striding down the sidewalk can do your heart good (although running is still considered super).

"To have an effect on heart disease, exercise has to be aerobic," says Mier Stampfer, M.D., assistant professor of medicine. "You can achieve a modest cardiovascular training effect with walking alone if you do it long enough and vigorously enough. You should walk at a brisk pace for a minimum of 20 to 30 minutes."

But once in a while is not enough. "If you're only walking for 20 minutes, you'd have to do it five days a week, maybe more," Dr. Stampfer says.

A "Benefishoil" Substance?

Newspapers have been stuffed to the gills recently with news about how fish and fish oil help the heart. Studies have shown that high levels of fish oil affect platelet function.

Platelets are elements in the blood that stick together to form a clot. Make them less "sticky," and your arteries are less likely to look like Manhattan at rush hour.

Some studies have also suggested that people who eat a lot of fish are at lower risk for developing heart disease. But the evidence is not yet conclusive. "I think it's promising and certainly worthy of research," says Dr. Stampfer. "But there're just not enough data yet to say for sure. The area is still under investigation."

Is all of this reason enough to turn to tuna in the meantime?

"We have to make a distinction between what we know scientifically and what we do while we're trying to learn those things," says Dr. Stampfer. "If you like fish and you want to eat more of it, it's partly a matter of taste, partly a matter of science."

Sack the Knife

Every year, approximately 200,000 men and women in the United States undergo a coronary-artery bypass operation. A new study suggests that as many as half of those operations could be safely avoided.

Thomas Graboys, M.D., assistant professor of medicine and attending cardiologist at the Brigham and Women's Hospital in Boston, and his colleagues studied 88 patients who were told by a cardiologist that they needed bypass surgery. All of the patients were referred for a second opinion. After a thorough evaluation, 74 of the patients were advised to continue medical therapy rather than have surgery. Sixty of those patients followed that advice.

None of those 60 patients died over the 28-month course of the study. What's more, 70 percent of them were still working full time and leading perfectly normal lives.

The results suggest that bypass operations are being done far too often. "It happens for three reasons," says Dr. Graboys. "First, the public views heart disease as a simple plumbing problem that surgery can easily fix. Second, there's a tremendous amount of fear of sudden death or heart attack once the patients hear they have heart disease. And third, we have a real density of heart surgeons who are trained in the techniques."

And while some doctors base the need for surgery on the degree of blockage in the coronary arteries, Dr. Graboys and others use different criteria. "What we realize now—and this is not just our study but a number of studies—is that the rate of having a heart attack or dying from heart disease is very low in people who have minimal symptoms, who have good, strong heart muscle, or who respond to medical therapy," says Dr. Graboys. "That's irrespective of whether they have narrowing of one, two, three, or four vessels. We have people who walk around with 95 percent narrowing of several vessels for years and years and years. And they have no symptoms and feel fine and do well. And the issue of bypass can either be deferred or postponed indefinitely."

In general, second opinions are reasonable for people who have stable symptoms, are feeling generally well, or

whose symptoms are controlled by medication, Dr. Graboys says. But it's important to make sure you really are getting a second opinion. "You don't necessarily get a second opinion from another cardiac surgeon," he says, "because cardiac surgeons operate. And you don't necessarily get one from the same cardiology group. There's a legitimate question whether you should even get a second opinion from the same hospital. You should probably look for a neutral, nonvested cardiologist."

In Dr. Graboys's study, medical therapy included diet and exercise programs and reduction of risk factors such as smoking, high blood pressure, and high cholesterol. But maximizing drug therapy was also an important component of treatment.

"There are now three classes of heart drugs: the calcium channel drugs, the beta-blockers and the nitrates," says Dr. Graboys. "They're made to work in different ways, and you can use these three basic groups together. It's called triple therapy." The drugs work together to reduce the workload on the heart, improve the blood supply, and prevent spasm of vessels that can cause angina, or chest pains.

Keeping track of three drugs may sound like complicated business. But the newer preparations are sufficiently long acting that some have to be taken only once or twice a day, Dr. Graboys says.

Aspirin for Your Aching Heart

With TV commercials now touting aspirin as a drug dear to your heart, a little clarification might be in order. Aspirin is now licensed by the Food and Drug Administration for use by people with unstable angina and people who have had a heart attack. "It's generally advisable that those people take aspirin regularly under a physician's supervision," says Dr. Stampfer. It is believed to inhibit platelets from sticking together, preventing blood clots that can cause a heart attack.

What makes aspirin therapy especially attractive is that just a little tab'll do ya. "One aspirin a day is actually far more than you need to reduce platelet aggregation," says

Dr. Stampfer. "One every other day, or even one baby aspirin a day, is enough." Taking a small dose or using enteric-coated aspirin can reduce the stomach irritation that aspirin sometimes causes.

The important point to remember is that aspirin is indicated only for people who have had a heart attack or who have unstable angina and are under a doctor's supervision. "There's no evidence available right now that would recommend that healthy people take aspirin to prevent heart attacks," says Dr. Stampfer. "That issue is currently under study and we should have an answer in perhaps a couple of years."

Straight Talk about Cigarettes, Coffee, and Alcohol

If someone you know is looking for encouragement to quit smoking, hit 'em with this: Most evidence supports the view that if you quit smoking, your risk for heart disease drops very rapidly and approaches that of someone who's never smoked. "We're not sure," says Dr. Stampfer, "but it's probably a matter of months or even days."

Smoking roughly doubles a person's risk of heart disease. In fact, in a study of over 120,000 women, the Nurses' Health Study, researchers found that smoking probably accounts for half the heart attacks in middle-aged women. "It's a somewhat ignored risk factor," says Dr. Stampfer. "Smoking actually kills more people from heart disease than it does from lung cancer." Unfortunately, a person's risk of lung cancer drops only gradually after quitting smoking.

What about coffee, which seems to have gotten a bad rap, at least with respect to its link to heart disease? Well, according to Dr. Stampfer, "the bulk of the evidence does not favor an association between moderate coffee intake and heart disease."

So where did the idea come from? Smokers tend to drink a lot of coffee. And smokers have higher rates of heart disease. "So when you look at the effect of coffee on the heart, you have to rule out the effect of smoking," says Dr.

Stampfer. "Once you do this, there's little evidence for an association between coffee and heart disease, except perhaps in the highest levels of intake."

Many people have heard that imbibing alcoholic beverages protects your heart. They may wonder, is it true, or is it just wishful drinking?

"Most studies continue to support the view that moderate alcohol intake is associated with a reduced risk of heart disease," says Dr. Stampfer. Alcohol's ability to raise the level of high-density lipoprotein (HDL) cholesterol—the beneficial kind—is the probable cause.

"The reduction in risk starts to become apparent at a level of one drink per day or even less," says Dr. Stampfer. "Risk continues to go down until you reach two or three drinks a day." After that, excessive alcohol use increases the risk of heart disease.

"I think, in general, an approach of moderation is sensible," says Dr. Stampfer. "There are a lot of ill effects from drinking, even among nonalcoholics. So I wouldn't recommend to somebody who hates to drink that he should drink as though it were medicine to lower risk. After all, you can lower your risk in other ways, too."

Change of Life, Change of Heart?

Women have turned to estrogen replacement therapy for years to relieve some of the unpleasant symptoms that can occur at menopause. But it may be helpful for something much more serious than hot flashes.

Graham Colditz, M.D., and his colleagues have been studying a group of 120,000 women. First they found that postmenopausal women who take estrogen have about half the heart attack risk of those who do not take estrogen.

Then in another study, they found that women who'd had both ovaries surgically removed (before menopause) and didn't take any replacement estrogen had double the risk of heart disease. Those who did take estrogen were at no greater risk than premenopausal women of the same age who had not had surgery.

"They're pretty powerful data," says Dr. Colditz, in-

structor in medicine. "The estrogen/heart disease association has been seen in a number of studies. Ours is by far the largest."

The most likely explanation for the findings is estrogen's effect on blood fats. Women taking estrogen have higher levels of HDL and lower levels of low-density lipoprotein (LDL) cholesterol—the artery-clogging kind.

Is the evidence considered solid enough to recommend the use of estrogen replacement therapy? "Yes, definitely," says Dr. Colditz. "At this stage I think the benefits outweigh the risks."

"In-Fat-Uated" with Cholesterol

Before you go on a heart-healthy diet, make sure you have your fats straight. If you think that cholesterol is the only villain in your diet, your effort will be doomed. "If you want to reduce your blood levels of cholesterol, it's more important to lower your intake of saturated fat," says Dr. Stampfer. "It's not enough to just give up eggs and a few things that have a lot of cholesterol. You have cut the saturated fat to lower the blood cholesterol levels." Doctors have known that for a long time, he says, but for some reason people focused on cholesterol and forgot about the rest.

And just as cholesterol has epitomized the "bad fat" in people's minds, polyunsaturated fats have gotten all the glory. But there's another kind of fat that helps the heart: monounsaturated fat—the kind found in olive oil.

We've known for decades that polyunsaturated fats tend to lower cholesterol levels. And it was believed that monounsaturates had no effect. "The current research is tending to challenge that," Dr. Stampfer says. New research shows that monounsaturates do lower cholesterol. What's more, research shows that they also raise HDL.

"I think it's interesting because it means that people can feel comfortable using monounsaturates," says Dr. Stampfer. "Basically it comes down to a reduction of saturated fat and perhaps partial replacement with polyunsaturates and monounsaturates."

Salt's Role Still Not Clear

Here's another possible fallacy that's been sprinkled around quite liberally: Salt causes high blood pressure. "In spite of all the research, the answer on salt is not really in," Dr. Stampfer says. "It's certainly clear that people who have hypertension should be on a low-salt diet. A lot of those people will experience a decline in their blood pressure. But as far as reducing salt to reduce the incidence of high blood pressure, we just don't know." Since the average American's salt intake is much higher than necessary, prudence dictates moderation.

The subject of salt continues to be controversial, and that in itself can be a problem. "I think its importance has probably been exaggerated to the point of distracting people from more important diet issues, such as fat," Dr. Stampfer says.

A Hostile Takeover of the Heart

You've probably heard that stress can be bad for your heart. But do you know which emotions are the real heartbreakers?

"It's a function of whether or not the sympathetic nervous system is activated by the stress," says Herbert Benson, M.D., associate professor of medicine and author of *Your Maximum Mind.* "It has to do with the so-called fight-or-flight response. When that occurs, blood pressure increases and more work is placed on the heart. In particular, anxiety and hostility seem to be most closely related to elevations in blood pressure."

People don't have to fall victim to their own bad temper, though. "Antistress measures are being used more and more in cardiology, both in prevention and in treatment," says Dr. Benson. "The techniques that elicit the 'relaxation response' are the cornerstone." The relaxation response is the capacity of the body to enter a peaceful state in which body metabolism, heart rate, breathing rate, and blood pressure are lowered. Those changes counteract the harmful effects of stress.

"There is now rather strong evidence that the relaxation response is effective in reducing blood pressure to the extent that stress might be causing it," says Dr. Benson. "After regular treatment, anxiety and hostility and anger tend to diminish. The extent of improvement in blood pressure seems to correlate rather well with the degree to which anxiety and hostility are alleviated."

There are scores of techniques that elicit the response: meditation, prayer, yoga, or various forms of exercise. And there are many audio tapes and books that teach how to do this.

Everyday Heartthrobs

Most people have experienced the feeling of their heart skipping a beat at some time. But some people's hearts beat a funky rhythm much of the time.

Many new drugs are commonly available to treat abnormal heart rhythms, but "the indications for treatment are really very few," says Dr. Graboys. Doctors now know that heart rhythm changes are common and that the majority of people who have them don't need treatment. Of course, it's important to check with your doctor to rule out a serious disturbance.

Cholesterol Countdown

Can exercise overrun the effects of a high-fat diet? It's a question often asked (in a hopeful tone) by those who would rather sweat than diet. After all, exercise is good for the heart and can even boost HDL levels.

That sounds reasonable, but it isn't necessarily so. "You can still have a high degree of atherosclerosis," says Dr. Stampfer. "You have to get your blood levels of cholesterol down." And the only way to know if that's happened is to have your cholesterol level checked.

The same is true for those who'd happily watch every morsel they eat rather than lace on a pair of sneakers. "You have to look at the net effect," Dr. Stampfer says. "If you achieve your dietary goals—low cholesterol level and a low LDL to HDL ratio—you put yourself into a low-risk

group even without exercise (although I think exercise is healthy anyway). But *you have to get your cholesterol checked* to see if it's working. Some people think they're being very careful about their diet and in fact they're not."

If a cholesterol test is a good idea, are regular exercise tests and EKGs even better?

"I'm not a proponent of routine exercise tests," says Dr. Graboys. "If someone has symptoms, then it's reasonable to do. But the problem is, if you take 500 middle-aged men and do exercise tests on all of them, you'll find that about 20 percent [100 men] will have some change in the rhythm of their heart. And as many as two-thirds of those will be what they call false-positives. So all of a sudden you've got perfectly healthy people who are now patients."

If you have a high number of risk factors, your doctor may recommend those tests. But for most people, it's unlikely to be worthwhile.

What Have You Got to Gain?

It's a question that begs to be answered before you embark on a change of lifestyle. Just what kind of payoff can you expect from a cholesterol-lowering diet?

It's an issue that's attracted some controversy lately. In a recent study, William C. Taylor, M.D., and his colleagues attempted to calculate the benefit in life expectancy that could be gained from a lifelong program of cholesterol reduction. They found that people who are at high risk could add months or even years to their life expectancy. But people at low risk might add only days or weeks. "Our results were taken as running counter to the prevailing wisdom," Dr. Taylor admits.

"The impact from smoking cessation and blood pressure control is vastly greater than the impact from dietary intervention to change the blood cholesterol level," he says. One reason that's true is because smoking and high blood pressure contribute to other diseases beside just heart disease. Another is that when somebody goes on a diet to change his or her cholesterol level, it might not change that much. In one study of 12,000 men, the average reduction achieved by diet was 6.7 percent.

That figure is just an average, however. "Some people go on a diet and their cholesterol may go down 10, 15, or even 20 percent," Dr. Taylor says. "I personally think it probably is prudent to go on a diet. I hope that people continue to do so. But I think they ought to do that with their eyes open. And I'd want them to talk to a health professional who can individualize the recommendations based on their own characteristics." Here again, your doctor can see if diet is working for you by checking your blood cholesterol level.

Diet or Drugs?

Diet is always the first line of defense against high blood cholesterol levels. But should that fail, there are a number of drugs that doctors can turn to that bring cholesterol down. Many doctors rely on them, but others are wary.

While drugs do lower cholesterol, most of the studies done so far have failed to show that they lower the death rate, too.

New and more effective drugs are getting a lot of attention, though. And the hope is that eventually they will be shown to lower the death rate. "I think in the next five years there'll be a whole host of these agents available that'll be essentially safe, taken once a day, and well tolerated," says Dr. Graboys. "And they'll help keep cholesterol down."

And that's good news, because recent reports show that reducing cholesterol in the blood may actually reverse the buildup of artery-clogging plaque. A disease process once regarded to be as inevitable as the march of time may be halted by diet or drugs, researchers are finding.

In a recent and much heralded study, researchers monitored 162 men with atherosclerosis. Their arteries were x-rayed before and after the two-year study. The x-rays showed clearly that cholesterol-lowering drugs and low-fat diets stopped the progression of the disease in many of the men. And in some of them, the blood vessels actually became *less* clogged. Several other studies have shown similar results. And many of these "regression" studies are currently under way and may soon confirm those findings.

"The data are fairly persuasive, though more studies are needed," says Dr. Stampfer. "Meanwhile, I think that the current data should give people a lot of encouragement."

CHAPTER 11

Speed Your Way to Recovery with Arginine

By Hans Fisher, Ph.D.

From detoxifying blood to mending wounds, this amino acid's healing virtues are just now being recognized.

The amino acid arginine was first discovered and isolated 100 years ago. It's one of the 20 amino acids that are the building blocks of protein. Until the 1970s, arginine (pronounced *AR-juh-neen*) was considered to be a nonessential amino acid, meaning that it was not required in the diet by people of all ages. Since then, however, its importance has been found to stretch far beyond its role in making proteins.

It's now known to be essential for growing children, and a supplementary need for arginine has been established for people with liver or kidney disease. Perhaps most exciting, though, is its newly discovered ability to speed healing.

A renowned physician/nutritionist, Sir David Cuthbertson, from Glasgow, Scotland, suggested some 20 years ago that the striking protein loss observed in patients with severe trauma, such as burns, arm or leg fractures, or major

surgery, might be avoided by providing carefully chosen amino acids in the diet. This suggestion contradicted common medical opinion at the time. It was then held that little could be done nutritionally to stop the body's heavy loss of protein.

The size of this protein loss is indeed staggering. Patients with multiple fractures, for example, have been known to lose the protein equivalent of the whole liver within nine days following the fractures. The protein loss from the body's organs can be so great that they can't perform their normal functions. And that can make recovery even more difficult.

Research Results

More than ten years ago, researchers at a laboratory at Rutgers University undertook the test of Sir David's theory. They knew that the scar tissue that forms during the healing process has a high arginine content and that arginine is needed for several other important purposes as well. So it may simply not be available in adequate amounts for this additional burden, even when the patient eats a balanced diet.

In laboratory animals with fractures, diets supplemented with extra arginine and glycine (another amino acid) reduced the loss of protein by 40 percent, the researchers found.

Within a year after the initial observation, researchers at Einstein Medical School in New York City confirmed and extended this work. They reported that following moderate surgery, patients who received an extra 15 grams of arginine per day had a 60 percent reduction in protein loss compared to patients who did not get the supplement. Further studies in lab animals have shown that arginine helps wounds heal faster and more completely.

One member of the Einstein research group suggested that arginine may influence the repair process not only through its role in scar tissue formation but also because it improves the immune response of the thymus gland. By preventing infection, it may aid wound healing.

A supplemental source of arginine has also been found

useful in people with certain liver disorders. When the liver isn't working properly, dangerously high levels of ammonia can accumulate. Arginine helps detoxify the ammonia. In some clinical studies with patients suffering from liver disease, arginine was shown to reduce high blood-ammonia levels and overcome the often associated coma. Arginine is currently being used in several foreign countries to treat liver disease. In this country, other amino acids are being tried with mixed success.

People who suffer from kidney disease are thought to be in special need of extra arginine, too, to compensate for dialysis and an inability to make enough of the amino acid.

Every movement we make requires the use of our muscles and necessitates energy to make those muscles contract. One of the important chemicals in muscle that helps provide the energy for these contractions is a substance called creatine. Creatine, in turn, is made from arginine.

Arginine is also involved in the transport and excretion of the element nitrogen, the distinguishing component of proteins and amino acids. Arginine helps the body get rid of the nitrogen that is freed when body proteins are broken down. That prevents toxic levels from building up. It does this by transforming the nitrogen into urea, which is the most important nitrogen-containing constituent of urine.

Arginine is also known to stimulate secretion of hormones from several endocrine glands. Its effects on growth-hormone secretion by the pituitary gland and insulin secretion by the pancreas are particularly striking. (The stimulation of growth hormone may contribute to arginine's effect on wound healing.) Why and how arginine stimulates hormone release is still not known, but it is thought to be a normal function in everyone.

There is some evidence that arginine supplementation can help men who are infertile but otherwise healthy. In one study, out of 178 men who were given 4 grams of arginine daily, 62 percent showed a significant improvement in sperm count. In a smaller clinical trial with 18 infertile men, though, there was no apparent benefit.

There is also evidence that arginine inhibits some of the cancer-forming capacity of various chemical agents. And studies have shown that it interferes with the growth of

Keen on Arginine

If you're looking to beef up your arginine intake, you may be pleased to know that it's found in other foods besides meat. You can see for yourself from the list below.

Food	Portion	Arginine (mg.)
Turkey breast, roasted	4 oz.	2,377
Lamb, roasted	4 oz.	2,242
Flounder, baked	4 oz.	2,184
Beef chuck, braised	4 oz.	2,149
Cod, broiled	4 oz.	2,130
Chicken, roasted with skin	½ breast	1,800
Salmon, baked	4 oz.	1,730
Bluefish, baked	4 oz.	1,684
Pumpkin seeds	¼ cup	1,683
Halibut, broiled	4 oz.	1,620
Swordfish, broiled	4 oz.	1,615
Crabmeat, steamed	½ cup	1,506
Salmon, pink, canned	½ cup	1,276
Tuna, canned	½ cup	1,211
Peanuts, dry-roasted	¼ cup	1,163
Chick-peas	½ cup	793
Filberts	¼ cup	737
Sunflower seeds	¼ cup	722
Lentils	½ cup	674
Cottage cheese, 1% fat	½ cup	638
Kidney beans, canned	½ cup	419
Peas	½ cup	408

SOURCES: Adapted from *Nutrients in Foods*, by Gilbert A. Leveille, Mary Ellen Zabik, and Karen J. Morgan (Cambridge, Mass.: The Nutrition Guild, 1983) and USDA Home Economics Research Report No. 4 (Washington, D.C.: U.S. Department of Agriculture).

tumors transplanted from one animal to another. This is, of course, very exciting, and researchers expect that much more work will be done to clarify the anti-cancer role of arginine.

The Need for Arginine

The body itself can make some arginine from other amino acids. The rest we must get from our diet. But scientists calculate that the amount of arginine in our diet (an average of 5,400 milligrams, or 5.4 grams per day) is just barely sufficient to meet the daily need for creatine synthesis. It follows that the amount of arginine in the diet may be insufficient for its other functions. And it's clear that under specific clinical situations, such as recovery from severe malnourishment, trauma, kidney disease, and some types of liver disease, arginine is needed in amounts beyond that supplied by ordinary diets or synthesized by the body.

It's easy to get more arginine in your diet. Meat, poultry, and fish are good sources, because they're high in protein and arginine is a component of protein. But strategically, legumes are even better. Although they're not as high in protein, a greater percentage of their protein is arginine (7 to 12 percent versus about 6 percent). Since most Americans already get more than enough protein, eating more legumes is a good way to increase your arginine intake. Peanuts and soybeans are especially rich sources. Seeds are a good source, too. See the table "Keen on Arginine" on page 84 for more food sources.

CHAPTER 12

Walk for the Health of It: A Diabetic's Guide

Exercise can help you lose weight and keep your blood sugar under control. With benefits like that, you may be able to reduce (or even eliminate) your medication.

Many diabetics have the power to diminish the effects of their disease. Exercise can give them that power. How?

First, exercise helps regulate blood sugar by tinkering with insulin sensitivity. In fact, some Type I (insulin-dependent) diabetics find that with regular, moderate exercise, they can reduce the amount of insulin they need. Second, the calorie-burning benefits of exercise offer a bonus for the diabetic. People with non-insulin-dependent diabetes can often reverse the course of their disease through diet, exercise, and weight loss. Finally, aerobic exercise, which promotes heart and lung health, is especially important, since diabetics are at increased risk for coronary heart disease.

"Brisk walking is an excellent exercise for diabetics in good shape," says Henry Dolger, M.D., former chief of the Diabetes Department at Mount Sinai Medical Center in New York City.

Not only does walking deliver all of the fitness benefits described above, but it's easy on the body and there is very little risk of serious injury.

Of course, check with your doctor before you begin your walking program. Not all diabetics will benefit from exercise, and in some cases exercise may be dangerous. After you get your doctor's approval, keep him or her informed of your fitness progress. As you exercise more and perhaps

lose weight, your medication needs may change. But only your physician can determine that.

Aim for High Frequency

Walking at least three to five times a week (doctors' common recommendation to maintain a healthy heart) is good advice for the diabetic. It seems that the positive effect exercise has on blood sugar regulation is quickly lost once exercise is discontinued. So map out your walking log and make every effort to stick with your program. If you do skip a workout or two, don't try to make it up by walking faster or twice as far. Vigorous exercise can cause a rise in blood sugar, especially in people who have insulin deficiency.

Non-insulin-dependent diabetics, 90 percent of whom are overweight, may do well to walk five to seven times a week. This may improve the rate of weight loss.

And whether you use insulin or not, be sure to check with your physician regarding how long you should walk at each workout.

Exercising at the same time each day—whether early in the morning, over the lunch hour, or after work—helps to develop a habit of regularity. For diabetics, the timing of exercise can also help control blood sugar levels, says Dr. Dolger. Non-insulin-dependent diabetics may benefit from exercising before meals. This helps regulate appetite and promote weight loss. On the other hand, insulin-dependent diabetics are ill advised to exercise on an empty stomach when blood sugar is low. They should plan their walks for an hour or so *after* a meal, Dr. Dolger explains, when blood sugar levels are reaching their peak.

The reason for this is that exercise can sometimes send blood sugar levels into a tailspin. And if you use insulin, you're more likely to experience this hypoglycemic (too-low blood sugar) reaction. So eat before you walk and always carry along a snack for emergency purposes. Talk with your doctor about how much exercise you can tolerate before you need to replenish your store of carbohydrates.

Pamper Your Feet

For diabetics, comfortable walking shoes and socks are not just important, they're essential, says Marc A. Brenner, D.P.M., director of the Institute of Diabetic Foot Research. A small blister or callus may be insignificant to most people. But irritation may be life- or limb-threatening to a diabetic. To complicate the matter, diabetics often have difficulty feeling irritations on their feet. They are also more prone to infections.

Dr. Brenner suggests that if you're diabetic, you seek out a professional shoe fitter when selecting your walking shoes. As daily precautions, powder your feet to keep them dry and check your shoes and socks for any foreign particles and rough spots. If, despite these precautions, you develop a blister or other type of irritation, consult a physician or a podiatrist immediately—no later than the next day.

Keep Your Cool

Diabetics should avoid temperature extremes, says Dr. Brenner. If the weather outside is too hot (over 80°F, with humidity above 70 percent) or too cold (below freezing, taking into account the wind chill), for comfort's sake, head for the nearest shopping mall. Many doctors recommend that their patients walk in these temperature-controlled environments. And many malls now welcome walkers with special programs.

Carry I.D.

Always carry identification. It should include your name, address, and phone number, as well as your physician's phone number and information on your medical condition and the medications you take. If your walking pants don't have pockets to hold your I.D., consider a fanny pack, a wrist wallet, or a small pouch that attaches to the instep of your walking shoe.

If there's a silver lining here, it's this: Often, a health problem like diabetes can motivate a person to embrace a

more healthful lifestyle, one that includes regular walks. The result is not only improved health but also enjoyment of life.

CHAPTER 13

Lower Your Blood Pressure Naturally

More doctors are suggesting changes in your eating habits as the first—and sometimes only—treatment for hypertension.

These days, many more doctors are offering patients with high blood pressure the option of nondrug treatments. They may also recommend exercise and relaxation techniques, but the emphasis is on permanent changes in the way you eat. "Research shows that modifying your eating habits really can work," says Cleaves Bennett, M.D., medical director of the Los Angeles InnerHealth Clinic and coauthor of *The Control Your High Blood Pressure Cookbook.*

"Dietary changes help some people avoid ever having to take blood pressure drugs, and they help others decrease their dosage," Dr. Bennett says. "And they can work for people who've had high blood pressure for years. But they need to be given a chance—two months minimum, and up to a year for people with severe high blood pressure. Both patient and doctor need to be committed to making the changes work." (And, of course, any changes, especially reductions in medication, should be made under medical supervision.)

So what items do Dr. Bennett and others put on their patients' shopping list, and why? And what do they tell their patients to avoid? Here are their suggestions, along with the latest research findings on nutrients that really work against high blood pressure.

Much Ado about Magnesium

What do buckwheat pancakes, almonds, and bananas have in common? They're all good sources of magnesium, a mineral that tempers both steel and blood vessels. "Magnesium is probably one of the most promising and least-used minerals when it comes to blood pressure control," says Burton Altura, M.D., Ph.D., a leading researcher.

One recent study, by Honolulu Heart Program researchers, clearly shows magnesium's importance in blood pressure control. The scientists examined 61 different factors in the diets of healthy older men. Magnesium came out on top, having the strongest link between high intake and low blood pressure (*American Journal of Clinical Nutrition).* Many mineral researchers think an average-size man should be getting about 420 to 475 milligrams of magnesium a day to make up for what he loses—and to help protect him from developing high blood pressure as he ages. That's about 125 to 150 milligrams a day more than most men get.

Stock up on beans and nuts to guarantee that you'll get plenty of magnesium. Whole grains, leafy greens, and many other fruits and vegetables are also good sources. Hard water can be a good source of many minerals, including magnesium.

The Calcium Connection

Only recently have researchers noted that some cheese and milk lovers seem to have lower blood pressure. Now they are pinpointing just who benefits from additional calcium.

"Additional calcium seems to work best for people who are hypertensive and salt sensitive," says Lawrence Resnick, M.D., of the Cardiovascular Center at New York

Hospital/Cornell Medical Center. These are people whose blood pressure goes up 5 percent or more when they switch from a low- to a high-salt diet. In a recent study, Dr. Resnick found that adding 2,000 milligrams a day of calcium to the high-salt diets of salt-sensitive people blunted salt's blood pressure-raising effects. One-third to one-half of all people with high blood pressure, and especially blacks and older people, are salt sensitive, Dr. Resnick says (*Journal of Hypertension*).

"The present study indicates that the more salt elevates blood pressure, the more calcium lowers it," Dr. Resnick says.

Low-fat dairy products are excellent sources of calcium. Other good calcium sources are sardines, salmon, leafy greens, and nuts.

Pick Up on Potassium

People already taking blood-pressure medicines know their doctors keep a careful watch on their potassium levels. Some drugs make the body excrete potassium.

But giving extra potassium to people with mildly elevated blood pressure can make pressure drop, sometimes dramatically, according to two new studies.

Researchers at Duke University in Durham, North Carolina, gave one group of hypertensives a large daily dose of potassium. Another group got harmless lookalike pills, or placebos. After two months, blood pressure in the potassium-supplemented group had dropped significantly. One subgroup in particular—blacks—had the biggest drop: Their blood pressure went down by almost 20 points. "Blacks may be particularly sensitive to the blood pressure-lowering effects of potassium," the researchers conclude (*Hypertension*).

In another study, Italian researchers used potassium with similar results. They noted that those patients with the highest salt intake seemed to benefit most from the extra potassium (*British Medical Journal*).

Potassium does help counteract sodium's negative effects, says George D. Webb, Ph.D., coauthor with Richard D. Moore, M.D., Ph.D., of *The K Factor.* "We suggest you

get about three times as much potassium in your diet as you do sodium," Dr. Webb says. To meet that ratio, most people need to cut their sodium intake to 2,000 milligrams or less a day. And they must make a conscious effort to eat more potassium-rich foods, such as baked potatoes, avocados, raisins, sardines, nuts, orange juice, winter squash, bananas, and whole grains.

Sock It to Salt

Perhaps you've already cut back on salt by not adding it to foods at the table or when you cook. That's good. It helps you cut down by about one-third. But today, many people get much of their salt from foods that have salt added during processing. Unfortunately, that comprises a long list. Cold cuts, canned meats, many frozen dinners and entrées, canned vegetables, cheeses (including cottage cheese), crackers, and pickled foods are top-heavy with salt. When shopping for prepared foods, check labels to find reduced-sodium varieties.

"Try to cut your salt intake at least in half, down to 2,000 milligrams a day or less," Dr. Webb suggests.

Good Fat, Bad Fat

Butter, oil, bacon—all the fats we eat affect blood pressure because they are used by our bodies to make hormones known as prostaglandins. Some prostaglandins lower blood pressure, and whether the body manufactures this kind depends on which "building materials" it has on hand.

There are two important things to remember when you're changing the fat content of your diet to try to lower your blood pressure.

First, keep your total fat intake low—ideally, less than 30 percent of your total calories, Dr. Webb says. That's most easily done by cutting back on butter, margarine, oils, hard cheeses, fatty meats, and other concentrated fat sources.

Second, get more than half of your fat as polyunsatu-

rates, monounsaturates, and omega-3 fatty acids. All those fats appear to have blood pressure-lowering effects. Among polyunsaturated oils, choose those high in linoleic acid—safflower and sunflower seed oils. (Linoleic acid is used to produce the pressure-lowering prostaglandins.) Get monounsaturated fats from tasty olive and peanut oils. Omega-3 fatty acids, the oils found in such fish as salmon and mackerel, and in shellfish and some vegetable oils (canola, or rapeseed, oil), also seem to reduce blood pressure, at least when these fats are substituted for saturated fats.

In one study, a special breed of rats that naturally develop high blood pressure was fed a diet high in fish oils. After two weeks, the older rats' blood pressure levels had dropped significantly, and the younger rats hadn't had the kind of blood pressure rise they normally experience (*Federation Proceedings*).

In another study, by West German researchers, men with mild high blood pressure who ate two cans of mackerel a day for two weeks had a significant drop in blood pressure. Cutting back to three cans of mackerel per week maintained that newly lowered pressure for eight months. Their pressure reverted to its original high level only when the men went back to their old diet, which was low in fish and high in cold cuts (*Atherosclerosis*).

Avoid Alcohol

Heavy drinkers have much higher blood pressure than those who drink less. And even moderate drinking can cause blood pressure to rise, a recent study from Australia shows.

The study matched blood pressure with alcohol intake in men who were being treated for high blood pressure. Normally, the men were moderate to heavy drinkers. For this study, they got free beer—25 bottles a week. For six weeks, they drank beer with a 5 percent alcohol content. Then, for another six weeks, they drank beer with a 0.9 alcohol content. When blood pressures during these two times were compared, averages were about five points lower during the low-alcohol weeks.

Lose Some Weight

Finally, if you've been uninspired to lose the pounds you want to, consider this: Losing weight is sometimes the *only* thing people need to do to drop their blood pressure to normal. And you don't necessarily have to lose it all! Losing even a third or half of your excess weight can have a tremendous impact on your blood pressure, Dr. Bennett says. Luckily, the same foods that help your blood pressure in other ways can help you lose weight, too.

CHAPTER 14
Dental Advances to Make You Grin

Ease the pain of routine checkups and the ugliness of tooth hardware with up-to-the-minute technology.

Okay, admit it. You can take on the Los Angeles freeway, ask your supervisor for a raise, and fix the kitchen sink yourself, but when it comes to getting that long-overdue dental work done, well . . . maybe next month. Or better yet, next year.

Welcome to the club. Up to 35 million other Americans have what the American Dental Association terms "dental anxiety." And, as a 1986 study showed, almost half of us haven't seen a dentist in over a year, even though many of us need attention.

If thoughts of the Drill, the Needle, or a mouth that (in your opinion) will look like a highway under construction have you less than excited about going to the dentist, there is good news.

A Shot at Comfort

Almost all of us appreciate the anesthetic that blissfully numbs us before procedures such as decay removal begin. But we could certainly do without the way it's delivered, as well as the numbness that lingers for hours after we leave the office. Well, the needle's still necessary, but the other vexation isn't.

"Intraligamental injection is a new way to send painkiller to nerves," says Roger Levin, D.D.S., president-elect of the Baltimore Academy of General Dentistry. "It uses a high-pressure syringe and an ultrathin needle that slides down the side of your tooth. The anesthetic can be sent right to where the nerve enters the tooth. This is more efficient than the old method, which could only place the painkiller in the gum surrounding the nerve."

When this new delivery method is coupled with a type of anesthetic called Xylocaine, the result is *instant* pain protection. Previously, the dentist had to wait about 10 minutes until the medication took effect before he or she could begin. "Patients feel much less anxious now because they don't have time to sit there dreading the drill," notes Dr. Levin. "And there's one other benefit: no numbness. You can go right back to work and give an important speech if you have to."

Swish Away Decay

When his practice received a new product called Caridex, Bruce Small, D.M.D., lecturer at the University of Medicine and Dentistry of New Jersey in Newark, performed a little experiment on about 100 of his patients.

He asked them each one question. "Would you be willing to pay more for a cavity-removal method that cut down on the amount of drilling I did and the amount of anesthesia I used?" With one exception, every patient said yes—and money was no object. (The lone dissenter wanted to know how *much* more.)

Dr. Small then introduced a new product that *dissolves* decay (in most cases with greatly reduced pain). For only a

little more money (about $5 per cavity), Caridex makes a big change in decay removal.

The device is simple: A heating unit and pump are attached to a tube; at the end of the tube is a pencil-like applicator tip. A warm chemical solution flows from the tip over your decay-invaded tooth. The active ingredient in the solution loosens the bonds that hold the molecules of decay together. Your dentist can then rub away the decay. (Healthy tooth and gum tissue are not affected by the chemical.)

"Caridex doesn't make the drill obsolete," explains Dr. Small. "But it significantly reduces the need for the drill and anesthesia. I'm using only half as much anesthesia as I did two years ago."

The great news: If your cavity is small and located on an easy-to-reach spot, you can probably escape the drill and the shot of painkiller altogether. About 10 percent of cavities can be treated this way.

The almost-as-great news: If your cavity is located where the Caridex tip can't reach—under a filling or between teeth, for example—your dentist can use the drill to start the job and then gently "rinse" away the decay that's closer to your nerve.

The Caridex method leads to better fillings, too. "When we use Caridex alone or in combination with the drill, we pretty much leave the healthy tooth alone. What's left after the decay's gone is a rough, Grand Canyonlike surface. The filling ends up with more tooth to 'grab onto' and so has greater bonding strength. In other words, the filling will last longer," says Dr. Small.

Caridex has no side effects. But if you have high blood pressure, you should know the solution contains sodium chloride. You might want to first clear the procedure with your regular doctor.

No-Show Fillings

A sad fact about cavities is that victimized teeth usually look worse after they're filled. It's a rare adult mouth that isn't sporting a collection of gold, dark gray, and silver fillings.

Enter porcelain onlays and white fillings, the new natural-looking dental materials for the appearance-conscious.

"There's no clinical reason to get your metal fillings taken out. Some people, however, are opting to have a mouthful of gold and silver restorations replaced," says Dr. Levin. "Others are choosing natural-looking fillings when old ones fall out, or when a new cavity shows up."

Porcelain onlays are used to restore fractured teeth or teeth with large cavities. They're an alternative to crowns and amalgam fillings (a silver and mercury mix).

In addition to looking more attractive than a silver filling, porcelain bonded to the tooth is much stronger. And placing an onlay doesn't require as much healthy tooth to be ground away, as must be done when inserting crowns. Your dentist simply bonds the porcelain into place with a special resin and then stains it to match the color of your other teeth. The total cost is much more than the cost of a silver filling but less than that of a crown.

White fillings are another appearance-preserving option. They cost far less than porcelain onlays but are still about 10 to 20 percent more than silver fillings.

White fillings are made from a bonding material called posterior composite resin, and they can also be color-matched to your other teeth. They are, however, not without their drawbacks. "White fillings won't last as long as silver and may need minor repairs," notes Dr. Levin. "Research is continuing, though, and these kinks will probably be worked out soon."

Brace Yourself

Crooked teeth are not the bane of teenagers only. More than half of all Americans could benefit from orthodontic treatment, either to look better or to have less painful, better functioning mouths.

If your teeth could use straightening but you just can't see yourself as a middle-aged "metal mouth," you might want to check out new braces you just can't *see,* period. One kind is sapphire braces: They're constructed of a clear, manmade version of the precious gem. Another alternative is ceramic braces.

"In my practice, I fit more adults with braces than children," says Michael Diamond, D.D.S., assistant professor of orthodontics at New York University College of Dentistry. "Almost every single adult opts for sapphire or ceramic. The sapphire is so transparent that from 4 to 5 feet away, only one thin wire is visible. From 10 feet or more, you can't see anything. The ceramic braces are not transparent, they're translucent. They're like a chameleon: They pick up the color of the tooth."

Invisible braces of a different sort came out a few years ago but failed miserably. They were made of plastic and weren't strong enough to do the job. Worse yet, they were easily stained by food and drinks. Sapphire and ceramic braces are stronger than plastic—as strong as their metal predecessors—and are impossible to stain.

You can expect the total cost for treatment with sapphire or ceramic braces to be about 20 percent more than you'd pay for the metal kind. But the invisibility factor may be just the thing to hedge any hesitation you may have about finally attaining straight, healthy teeth. And "sapphire mouth" almost sounds like a compliment!

PART IV: UPDATE ON CANCER

CHAPTER 15

How Close Are We to a Cancer-Free Future?

Experts can't agree—or even say if medicine is doing all that much. For now, hope lies in prevention, not treatment.

Will there be a cure for cancer in your lifetime? Will there be a cure for cancer in *anyone's* lifetime?

There are questions that scientists currently find themselves in something of a civil war trying to answer. In a shot recently heard around the medical world, former National Cancer Insitute (NCI) staff member John C. Bailar III, M.D., Ph.D., accused the NCI's progress reports of being not just exaggerated but also misleading and possibly even counterproductive to the work that remains to be done.

"We have had very little success in reducing overall cancer death rates or incidence rates, or in improving case survival rates," Dr. Bailar stated in his now legendary attack. "To the extent that these measures embody national targets or goals, we are losing the war against cancer."

Dr. Bailar went on to call the NCI's plan of cutting cancer

deaths in half by the year 2000 "not only unattainable but so far from reality as to cast doubt on the credibility of NCI in other matters. If we take the beginning of the modern era of cancer research to be the early 1950s, we have had 35 years of unfulfilled promises."

Not content with harsh words, Dr. Bailar bolstered his attack with hard facts—these chilling numbers.

- The cancer mortality death rate per 100,000 was up from 162.2 in 1975 to 170.7 in 1984.
- The cancer incidence rate per 100,000 was up from 330.5 in 1975 to 351.8 in 1984.
- The five-year relative case survival rate has remained essentially unchanged since 1976.

"No broad cancer research program can be labeled successful unless it has an impact on the basic overall death rate," Dr. Bailar concluded in his *Issues in Science and Technology* report. "If we cannot reduce the age-adjusted death rate for all cancers combined, we have failed in our primary purpose."

Too Simple a View

What leg could the NCI possibly find to stand on against Dr. Bailar's well-armed revolt?

"Dr. Bailar's argument is based on a very limited view of the figures," claims NCI staff member Gregory Curt, M.D. "As a physician who works with cancer patients every day, I can tell you that in diagnosis as well as treatment, we have far more available to us today than we did 30 years ago, or even 5 years ago. Dr. Bailar's argument misses the trees for the forest. He has not been close enough to cancer treatment on a doctor-to-patient basis to feel the impact that our progress against this difficult disease has been making."

What's more, Dr. Bailar fails to give credit for gains cancer research has helped scientists make in other areas—in the fight against AIDS, for example, plus other viral and genetic disorders. So say the director of the NCI, Vincent T. Devita, Jr., M.D., and branch chief Edward J. Sondik, M.D.

"Many of the advances in molecular genetics we herald

today can be traced to the infusion of resources from NCI-sponsored research programs," Dr. Devita and Dr. Sondik say. "We make no apologies to anyone for this investment and point proudly to these achievements in fundamental science."

Dr. Bailar's accusations also are based on figures that are old, claim the two NCI doctors. The impact of many recent advances "has not yet been felt nationwide," they say. "The advances are too recent to be felt beyond the population captured in the clinical trials."

Dr. Bailar Responds

With regard to Dr. Curt's comments, Dr. Bailar says, "Dr. Curt has not explained why cancer death rate and cancer incidence rates are still going up."

To Dr. Devita and Dr. Sondik, Dr. Bailar responds, "Substantial credit is indeed due for the many spin-off benefits from our national effort against cancer. But they do not make up for our failure to attain the real objective: control of cancer."

And regarding recent advances, Dr. Bailar feels that "advances in cancer research are of no benefit to the general public unless and until they show up in the statistics for that same general public. Cancer death rates through October 1987—the most recent month available—still show no improvement."

Areas of Agreement

But perhaps the real story in all this lies in the areas in which Dr. Bailar and the NCI find themselves in agreement. Both say that more emphasis must be put on *prevention* of cancer, that early diagnosis is the key to successful treatment, and that the disease, unfortunately, has turned out to be far more of a monster than anyone could have imagined when research started over 35 years ago.

Prevention

"In research as well as in our message to the public, our efforts must be refocused toward prevention of this very

complex disease," Dr. Bailar says. "I do not say this out of any blind conviction that prevention is always better in principle than treatment. Treatment, had it worked, would have been better, and certainly easier. And there is no guarantee that prevention will work, either. Much of the research has not yet been done. If we can find ways to prevent cancer, prevention is going to require substantial changes in such things as our personal habits, very expensive measures to clean up the environment and the workplace, and adoption of new ways to build houses and modify existing ones. Cancer *treatment* must come to be seen as a second line of defense."

And the cancer establishment agrees. "Dr. Bailar's premise that prevention is the cornerstone of cancer control is correct," says Lewis H. Kuller, Ph.D., of the Department of Epidemiology at the University of Pittsburgh. "Half of the reduction in mortality we see for the year 2000 can be achieved by effective prevention," add Dr. Devita and Dr. Sondik.

Effects of the NCI's influence in encouraging over 40 million people to quit smoking since the Surgeon General's report 22 years ago are already apparent, Dr. Devita points out. Lung cancer in white males, for example, has begun to head downward for the first time in 50 years, and the NCI expects to see similar declines in other cancers since it has demonstrated the connections between asbestos and lung cancer, sun exposure and melanoma, and chlorinated water and bladder cancer.

Early Diagnosis

"My comments about lack of progress are in no way an argument against the earliest possible diagnosis and the best possible treatment of cancer," Dr. Bailar agrees. "Modern medicine already has much to offer to virtually every cancer patient, for palliation [relief of symptoms] if not always for cure."

"The sooner a cancer is found, the better," Dr. Curt says. "The disease by its very nature is one that becomes harder to treat as its dominance of bodily systems begins to increase. For anyone over the age of 40, we strongly recommend a schedule of regular checkups."

The Complexity of the Disease

It's never comforting to see turmoil between the powers that be, especially when the turmoil centers on something as potentially relevant as cancer. And yet, in all fairness to the warring parties, there would have been no division in the first place had cancer not turned out to be such a confounding foe.

"The more we've learned about cancer, the more we've realized we need to know," says Dr. Curt. "Not only are there literally hundreds of different types of cancer cells, but the cancer cell by its very nature has the ability to mutate spontaneously and hence change in ways that can make it suddenly resistant to treatments that had been working. This is why many cancers are treated in a variety of ways simultaneously. We're literally trying to outsmart the cancer cells' adaptive abilities."

All the more reason to adhere to a schedule of regular checkups, and to consider prevention cancer weapon number one.

CHAPTER 16

Is Calcium a Cancer Preventer?

By Cedric Garland, Ph.D., and Frank Garland, Ph.D.

How two California scientists looked at a map and (literally) saw the light.

EDITOR'S NOTE: Medical researchers have yet to agree on the causes of most common cancers. Many factors, including excess fat, fiber deficiency, alcohol intake, and other lifestyle components are currently being investigated and

debated. This chapter presents the theoretical evidence for one particularly intriguing diet/cancer link.

Our investigation began on a summer afternoon in 1979. We were sitting in a lecture hall at the Johns Hopkins University, where Cedric was a faculty member and Frank a graduate student. We were viewing a presentation of maps showing the rates of various cancers for each of the 3,056 counties in the United States, newly computed by Dr. T. J. Mason and his colleagues of the National Cancer Institute. On each map, the parts of the country with high rates were darkly colored, and areas with the lowest rates were white.

Most of the maps showed a random, shotgunlike pattern of light and dark. But two maps—one of breast cancer and one of intestinal cancer—struck us with their startling geographic pattern. Although we didn't know it then, this was to be the beginning of an unraveling of an epidemiologic mystery.

It looked as if someone had drawn a heavy line along the 40th parallel—through the middle of California and the tops of Arizona, New Mexico, Texas, Tennessee, and the Carolinas. Virtually all the places with high breast and intestinal cancer mortality rates were north of this line, and all those with low rates were south of it. The white low-cancer areas were far more frequent in the Sun Belt. For example, most of southern California and Arizona was white, as was New Mexico. The dark areas were located in the northern half of the country, particularly in the Northeast.

Cedric had a flash of inspiration. Could the cancer rates for intestinal and breast cancer be connected somehow with sunlight? Our first step in answering the question was to try to eliminate other possible explanations for the geographic differences. One such possibility involved food. Both fiber-containing vegetables and red meat had been strongly suggested as influences in the occurrence of colon cancer—fiber as a food that helped to prevent the disease, and fat and red meat increasing its likelihood.

Fat had been strongly suggested as a cause of breast

cancer as well. Perhaps eating patterns were different in various parts of the United States.

We obtained dietary consumption patterns for the nation from a survey conducted by the U. S. Department of Agriculture. The survey told us that food consumption is remarkably similar throughout the United States, including intake of fruits, vegetables, fats, and red meat. Supermarkets and fast-food restaurants have standardized American eating habits. So geographic differences in food consumption didn't exist to explain the vast differences in breast and intestinal cancer rates across the country.

Our next step was to look at all the available evidence to test the theory. We looked at patterns of cancer and death rates from around the world, searching for clues related to sunlight and other causes. One of the first observations we made was that the death rate from breast cancer was higher in cities than in rural communities at the same latitude. We guessed that people in big cities at any latitude were deprived of vitamin D as adults due to air pollution and urban lifestyles.

The Role of Sunshine

What was the significance of sunlight with regard to cancer rates? Sunlight reacts with cholesterol inside and on the surface of the skin to create vitamin D. Vitamin D helps the body absorb calcium. Here's how it works.

Three hormones regulate calcium in the body. Only one—vitamin D—is to some extent under our control. Vitamin D is the only vitamin that has two sources. It is present in a few foods, such as fortified milk and some kinds of fish. But what makes vitamin D so unique is that it's also made when the skin is exposed to sunlight. Sunshine activates the cholesterol on the skin, creating provitamin-D. This is transported to the liver and kidneys in sequence, where each adds a molecule to it. The final product is vitamin D, which is transported to the small intestine, where it directs the cells lining the intestine to produce a calcium-binding protein. This protein then lies in wait, ready to yank in any unsuspecting calcium coming

through the intestine. Once hooked, the calcium is carried everywhere in the body it is needed, including the breast and the rest of the intestine. Without vitamin D, most of the calcium is cast off, completely unused.

What is the relationship between calcium and cancer? Calcium carries messages, through bridges called tight junctions, between the cells of body tissues. If calcium levels drop too low, cells can't communicate efficiently. The tissue becomes disorganized. This sets the stage for cancer.

The Western Electric Study

In 1984, an opportunity arose to test the effects of dietary vitamin D and calcium on intestinal cancer in a group of 1,954 men. The men were employed by the Western Electric Company in a telephone-assembly plant near Chicago. They had filled out dietary questionnaires during 1957 and 1958 and had been followed carefully for occurrence of heart disease and cancer by a distinguished group of scientists, including Dr. Richard Shekelle, Arthur Rossof, Oglesby Paul, and Jeremiah Stamler.

Our friends and colleagues Dr. Michael Criqui and Dr. Elizabeth Barrett-Connor of the University of California at San Diego, Department of Community and Family Medicine, met Dr. Shekelle at an educational conference on heart disease epidemiology. Both Dr. Criqui and Dr. Barrett-Connor mentioned our theory to Dr. Shekelle and suggested that it could be tested using the study that Dr. Shekelle's group in Chicago had begun years before. Dr. Shekelle agreed, and we began the analyses.

The study, which we coauthored with Dr. Barrett-Connor, Dr. Criqui, Dr. Shekelle, and his colleagues Rossof and Paul, was published in the *Lancet* on February 9, 1985. Dietary histories were collected at the beginning of the study, *before* any disease occurred. The participants cooperated faithfully during the next 19 years, and all but three of the men remained in the study to the end.

Intestinal cancer takes about 20 years to develop. We knew that patterns of intestinal cancer linked to foods would be evident, since 20 years had passed since the

study began. Diet histories for the study had been collected by nutritionists to precisely measure the quantities of food eaten during the month before the interviews. Information on the foods the men ate and their intake of vitamins and other nutrients was calculated and stored for later analysis. At the end of the period, 49 of the men had developed intestinal cancer and 1,372 men were free of cancer.

We found that men who developed intestinal cancer were a little heavier than those who did not, but they consumed only a few more calories than those free of cancer. A typical American high fat intake (43 percent of the men's calories were from fat) was present in both groups. The two groups ate virtually identical amounts of animal and vegetable protein and carbohydrates. There were no significant differences in intake of saturated or unsaturated fats, dietary cholesterol, minerals (except calcium), and most vitamins. The intake of alcohol differed slightly: Heavier drinkers had slightly higher risk of intestinal cancer.

Much to our excitement, our findings showed that the men who developed intestinal cancer differed from those who did not in only two respects—they ate far fewer foods containing vitamin D and calcium. Men who took in calcium and vitamin D equivalent to 4½ glasses of nonfat milk per day had only about *one-third* the risk of intestinal cancer.

The men in the lowest-intake group took in less than the amount of vitamin D in an ordinary glass of vitamin-D-fortified milk (100 international units) per day, while the men in the highest-intake group took in the amount of vitamin D in three or four glasses of milk. The men who had the lowest intake of vitamin D developed about twice as much intestinal cancer as those who had the highest intake.

There was a threshold effect at 150 international units of vitamin D—the amount in 1½ glasses of milk. The threshold effect means there was no additional decrease in risk of intestinal cancer for men who consumed more than 150 international units of vitamin D per day.

Men who took in the lowest amount of calcium (less than 315 milligrams per day, or the amount of calcium in

1½ glasses of milk) had more than three times as much intestinal cancer as men who had the highest intake (1,200 milligrams or more per day, or the amount of calcium in 4½ glasses of milk). There was no threshold for the benefit of calcium. This means that we do not know the upper limit of protection that calcium can provide. The more calcium the men took in, the lower the risk they had.

The Laboratory Test

Cedric was invited to the Memorial Sloan-Kettering Cancer Center in New York to present these findings, where the results were warmly received.

Dr. Martin Lipkin and Dr. Harold Newmark of Memorial Sloan-Kettering Cancer Center were studying New Yorkers who were at high risk of intestinal cancer because of a strong family tendency to develop the disease. They designed a study to see what effect calcium might have on the tissue of the intestinal tracts of these people. They chose a dose of calcium that was about the same as the one we found to be associated with the lowest risk of cancer in our *Lancet* study of Chicago men.

The Memorial researchers discovered that these high-risk people, before taking calcium, had an unusually high rate of cell division in the intestine. During the test, these people took calcium at a dose of 1,250 milligrams per day, in the form of calcium carbonate. After two or three months of the dietary supplements, their intestinal cells stopped dividing at the abnormally high rate and adopted a rate of cell division typical of people at ordinary risk of intestinal cancer.

In other words, the clinical test performed at Memorial Sloan-Kettering verified our predictions of the effect of calcium on cancer growth at the microscopic level.

A Curious Exception

There was still one exception to our general findings about the connection between sunlight, calcium, and cancer. That exception was one that had been drummed into us by Dr. Abraham Lilienfeld at Johns Hopkins University.

"Breast cancer is almost nonexistent in Japanese women," he would say, "and we have no good explanation. Perhaps someone in this room will discover why."

Most residents of Japan live from 33 to 45 degrees north of the equator, a region with only moderate sunlight. The amount of sunlight reaching Japan is associated almost everywhere else in the world with high rates of breast and intestinal cancer.

But the rate of these cancers in Japan is very low—about 5 per 100,000. By comparison, other areas at the same latitude, such as San Francisco and Connecticut, have rates more than five times as high.

We felt that Japan was the odd case, the final telling clue. The meaning of the clue was first discovered 200 years before, although until our research no one connected the findings with breast cancer. It involved immunity to a disease in Japan that was then causing severely malformed bones in English children. The disease, rickets, was so common in London that it was called the English Disease. It first appeared when the English began burning wood and coal on a grand scale in London. As increasing amounts of ash from the wood and coal rose into the atmosphere, the pollution became so bad that it blocked London's sunlight.

With industrialization and urban pollution came bowlegs, knock-knees, and deformities of the chests and pelvises of infants and children. The disease became so troublesome in England that one physician traveled to Japan to find out why the disease was so rare in that country.

What he found was a population virtually free of rickets, and people who ate a diet loaded with fish.

This aspect of the Japanese diet, which to this day includes huge amounts of fish, suggested a cure for rickets to that early epidemiologist. It now suggests to us the reason the rates of breast and colon cancer were so low in Japan. Fish is loaded with vitamin D. Although the Japanese do not receive a great deal of sunlight, their *diet* provides the vitamin D their bodies need to help absorb calcium and prevent breast and colon cancer. This was the missing link, the exception, that reconfirmed our theories about vitamin D, sunshine, calcium, and cancer.

The connection between calcium and cancer had been confirmed. We found but one more way in which calcium is essential to health.

How Much Vitamin D Is Enough?

People who live in areas that receive a great deal of sunlight need *less* dietary vitamin D, because their bodies produce more vitamin D from the sun. People in northern and in heavily polluted areas need *more* calcium and vitamin D because of the lack of sufficient vitamin D-producing sunlight. The amount of calcium and vitamin D a person needs, therefore, varies.

The present recommended daily intake of vitamin D in most countries is 200 to 400 international units per day, which is the amount in two to four 8-ounce glasses of fortified milk. Similar amounts of vitamin D are available from ordinary servings of salmon or other kinds of fish.

We don't recommend increasing the amount of sunlight you receive by exposing yourself for longer periods of time to direct sunlight. People who live in northern climates are usually not well adapted to strong sunlight and run a considerable chance of developing skin cancer due to overexposure. For this reason, we suggest moderate to little intentional direct exposure to the sun, particularly from 10:00 A.M. to 2:00 P.M. The same wavelength of light that stimulates production of vitamin D in the skin, UV-B, increases the risk of skin cancer.

CHAPTER 17
"If You Want to Live . . . Love and Laugh!"

Yale surgeon Bernard S. Siegel, M.D., reveals his unorthodox anti-cancer theory in an exclusive interview.

Spontaneous remission: It's medicine's explanation for the inexplicable—when cancer or another serious disease appears to improve or disappear "by itself." We tend to think of it as a favorable accident of fate—a modern-day miracle of sorts. But Dr. Bernie Siegel thinks differently.

Dr. Siegel, who is the author of the book *Love, Medicine and Miracles,* which was on the *New York Times* best-seller list for months, says, "Patients who get well when they're not supposed to are not having accidents or miracles or spontaneous remissions. They're experiencing self-induced healing."

As attending surgeon at Yale/New Haven Hospital and clinical professor of surgery at Yale Medical School, Dr. Siegel is not only affiliated with one of the nation's leading medical schools, he practices in a field that's widely regarded as the least humanistic of all medical specialties. Yet he takes an unconventional approach. He hugs his patients and insists that they call him Bernie. His diagnostic tools include crayons, with which he asks patients to draw pictures of their illness. And in his operating room, the clang of surgical instruments is drowned out by soothing music.

Beneath these practices lies a "natural healing" philosophy. Dr. Siegel believes, for example, that medical treatment is only as effective as the patient's unconscious mind allows, and that a combination of stress reduction, conflict

resolution, and positive reinforcement can stimulate the immune system and allow healing to take place.

In the medical world, Dr. Siegel's views are unorthodox and tough to test. But he maintains that his clinical experience bears him out.

In an exclusive interview, Dr. Siegel was asked why he believes that psychological and emotional factors can affect our vulnerability to disease and what measures might improve our chances for recovery.

Q. *How did you come to develop such an unorthodox approach to healing?*

A. I had become disturbed and unhappy in my role as a surgeon. My problem was in dealing with my feelings while being told that doctors don't touch people. They don't get involved with their patients' personal problems. So in an attempt to make myself happier as a doctor, I went to workshops. At one I met some of my own patients. They said to me, "Look, you're a good doctor. You listen to us and support us. But what are we supposed to do *between* office visits?"

So I set up group sessions to help them. As I saw people learning how to live with their illnesses, I saw them gaining incredible control over their wellness. I saw people dealing with conflict in their lives and then, suddenly, having their cancer shrink or disappear. These were things I had never seen before. I was astonished. And as a physician, I felt uncomfortable with it. They were getting better and I hadn't lifted a finger.

Q. *Why did you feel uncomfortable that people were getting well?*

A. You have to remember that medicine is failure oriented. We deal only with patients who *don't* get well. Those who get well when they're not supposed to are told not to return. These are patients we really ought to be studying. Instead we treat them as medical anomalies.

I got a note from an oncologist the other day. It said, "Roz is doing *amazingly* well. Her cancer is gone." I know Roz. I know why her cancer disappeared. Roz was sent to a nursing home to die. She hated it there. They weren't

attending to her needs. So, instead of passively accepting her situation, she stood up and led a revolution in the nursing home. She returned home and her cancer went away.

Q. *You make it sound easy. Is it?*

A. It's not easy at all. If I said to patients, you have two choices if you want to get well—you can change your lifestyle or have an operation—the majority would say, "Operate. It hurts less."

Generally, I find that about 15 to 20 percent of all people with chronic or catastrophic illness are truly exceptional—survivors. They are people who, when confronted with illness, are willing to take responsibility for it and redirect their lives accordingly. They are also willing to participate in their own recovery—to join with the doctor and become a healing team and to seek out all available resources to give themselves the best chance for getting well.

The majority of people—50 to 60 percent—are content to sit back and let their doctors direct their treatment. Their attitude is, "You're the doctor: Take care of me." Then there's another 20 percent who are happy to die because their lives are in shambles. For them, cancer is a very easy way out.

Q. *Are you saying that surviving cancer has as much to do with attitude as the extent of the disease?*

A. Yes, absolutely. I can usually determine where a person stands by asking four simple questions: (1) Do you want to live to be 100? This gives me an idea whether someone feels in control of his life and looks forward to the future. (2) What does your disease mean to you? This tells me if the person sees the disease as a challenge to overcome or as an overwhelming obstacle—a death sentence. (3) Why do you need this illness? This tells me whether the disease serves some psychological or emotional purpose. Is it a cry for love and nurturing? Or is it a signal from the body that you need some time off—from a job or from responsibilities? (4) What happened in the year or two before you got sick? This lets the patient know how he may have participated in his own illness. About 90 percent of

the cancer patients I see experienced significant change in their lives within the previous year or two. It may have been very devastating, like the death of a child or spouse—but it could also have been a positive change, such as moving to a new house, having a baby, or changing jobs.

Q. *But why is it that many people change jobs and move to new homes and don't get sick?*

A. Generally, it has a lot to do with meeting your own needs, expressing your feelings, learning to say no without guilt. Now, I'm not suggesting that people blame themselves for an illness. Rather, they should see the illness as a message to redirect their life accordingly—to resolve conflicts with other people, express anger and resentment and other negative emotions they've been bottling up inside, to begin looking out for their own needs. And, in so doing, the immune system becomes stimulated and healing takes place.

Learning to let go of negative emotions is key. The person who smiles on the outside and is hurting on the inside is not dealing with himself or his life. All his "live" mechanisms are told to stop working. By "live" mechanisms I mean endorphins, immune globulins, white blood cells, and other factors.

Doctors see examples of this every day. You are making rounds at the hospital and you ask a patient how she's doing and she says, "Fine." But you know she's not doing fine. Her husband ran off with another woman. Her son is on drugs. And she has cancer. But still she says, "Fine."

When I find a person who answers, "Lousy," I say, "That's wonderful! You want to get better so you're dealing with the truth. If your mind and body are feeling lousy and you're relating to that, you'll ask for help."

Q. *So what do you suggest that people do to help their "live" mechanisms work for them?*

A. Essentially, we must learn to open the lines of mind/body communication—to send "live" messages to the body. There are two ways to communicate these. One is through emotions. I tell patients, "If you want to die, stay depressed; if you want to live, then love and laugh." Posi-

tive emotions like love, acceptance, and forgiveness stimulate the immune system.

The second way to send "live" messages is through images—by visualizing the healing process taking place in your body. Think of your cancer cells as morsels of food and your white blood cells as birds, kittens, or Pac-Man—any food-eating image you feel comfortable with. Then close your eyes, quiet your mind, and imagine your white blood cells gobbling up the cancer cells. The more they eat, the stronger you become. In this way, the disease becomes a source of personal strength.

One caution: Some researchers suggest that cancer patients visualize aggressive white blood cells *attacking* or *killing* the cancer cells in their bodies. I think the majority of people have difficulty reconciling attack images in a healing context.

Q. *But isn't that the general perception of cancer—that it is an enemy that has somehow invaded the body?*

A. Yes. That's a problem. The ultimate example is a Quaker who refused treatment because his oncologist said, "Take this and it will kill your cancer." The patient said, "I don't kill anything," and walked out.

For most people, the rejection takes place at the subconscious or unconscious level. Their body simply refuses to respond to treatment. For example, I asked a child patient who was first brought to me because she wasn't responding to chemotherapy to draw a picture of herself receiving the treatment. In her picture, she's got a spear in her hand, supposedly to kill the cancer, but it's pointed in the wrong direction. Her cancer cells are crying, "Help me." The patient's *perception* of her treatment hampered her body's ability to respond favorably to it.

Q. *You're not suggesting that these mental exercises can be used as an alternative to conventional cancer treatments such as chemotherapy or surgery, are you?*

A. Certainly not! I am a surgeon, remember. I know that surgery and chemotherapy and radiation therapy can work wonders. I also know that the right attitude can sometimes help those treatments work even better.

You can preprogram yourself to respond favorably to chemotherapy or another treatment using a visualization technique similar to one athletes use to prepare for a race. By mentally rehearsing the event with a positive outcome, your body will get the message as to how it should respond in real life. Close your eyes and picture yourself sitting comfortably in a chair and having the chemotherapy or other treatment. Feel the cancer shrinking and your strength returning. After the treatment you feel good—even energized. To be effective, repeat this visualization maybe 100 times before starting the therapy.

Of course, the best way to ensure the effectiveness of any treatment is to know that the decision to have that treatment is yours. Find a physician who's willing to talk with you and lend support. Explore all your options together. Then choose the course of treatment you want. People who share and talk with their physicians—and who choose their therapies for positive reasons—have maybe one-fourth to one-tenth the side effects of people who just silently submit to treatment because their doctors or spouses told them they *had* to have it.

Q. *Do you find that today's doctors generally welcome this kind of team approach to healing?*

A. Some do. Some obviously still prefer submissive, nonquestioning patients. My advice is, don't worry if your doctor thinks you're being too assertive or inquisitive. In fact, consider it a healthy sign. Studies have shown that the patients physicians say are the biggest pests are the ones whose immune systems are the most active. They are the long-term survivors. The patients physicians say are wonderful—submissive and unquestioning—are the ones who are dying. So I tell people, develop a bad relationship with your doctor—based on *his* definition of bad. "Bad" by his standards is "good" by yours.

Q. *Can you give us some tips on how to be "bad" patients?*

A. Be assertive. Ask questions. Try calling your doctor by his or her first name. Give him a hug. The goal is, get to be a person—not just a disease—to that doctor. Approaching your doctor on a more human level causes him to

confront you in a different way—to treat you like a person with feelings and concerns.

Q. *What's the most important contribution a doctor can make to the recovery of a patient?*

A. I think there are two: The first is to give the patient control over his or her own treatment. The second is to offer hope.

If there's one thing I learned from my years of working with cancer patients, it's that there is no such thing as false hope. Hope is real and physiological. It's something I feel perfectly comfortable giving people—no matter what their situation. I know people are alive today because I said to them, "You don't have to die."

If statistics say that nine out of ten people die from this disease, many physicians will tell their patients, "The odds are against you. Prepare to die." I tell my patients, "You can be the one who gets well. Let's teach you how." I'm not guaranteeing immortality. I'm asking them if they want to learn how to live.

Q. *What's the best piece of advice you can give a cancer patient?*

A. The best piece of advice I give to anybody is *live each day as if it were your last.* That's not to say go rob a bank or spend your family savings. I'm talking from a spiritual standpoint. Make yourself happy. Resolve your conflicts. Get things off your chest. Find that peace of mind, that clear conscience. I guarantee, you'll wake up the next morning feeling so good, you won't want to die.

CHAPTER 18

The Male Manual of Cancer Prevention

A review of risk factors, diagnostic tests, and the best lifestyle strategies.

AIDS may have stolen the spotlight and heart disease may remain number one, but more than 20 percent of deaths in American men are caused by cancer—a statistic that is all the more chilling for being essentially unchanged despite 35 years of concentrated cancer research.

So do we drink up, light up, and let our genetic chips fall where they may?

"Absolutely not," says National Cancer Institute staff member Gregory Curt, M.D. "It would be a mistake not to take action, given what we know now about cancer."

John C. Bailar III, M.D., Ph.D., professor of epidemiology and biostatistics at McGill University in Montreal, agrees. "If our 35 years of research have taught us anything, it's that cancer is a disease more effectively prevented than cured."

Studies now suggest that as many as two-thirds of all cancers may be due, at least in part, to lifestyle factors—smoking, food abuse, environmental assaults. These, rather than genetic tendencies or simple bad luck, appear to be the instigating force in the vast majority of cancer occurrences. That being the case, here's a roundup of the male cancers that doctors currently consider the most preventable.

Lung Cancer

Estimated cases in 1987: 99,000; estimated deaths: 92,000.**

Despite small declines in recent years, cancer of the

*All figures given are for American men.

lungs continues to kill more than any other form of malignancy. It also remains one of the least curable cancers, sparing only 5 to 10 percent of its victims. As many as 90 percent of all cases of lung cancer may be *preventable,* however, and therein lies the real tragedy. Smoking remains the number one cause of lung cancer, increasing odds of the disease by as much as 25 times. Cessation of smoking, however, cuts odds of contracting lung cancer by 50 percent in 5 years and brings risks back down to those of a nonsmoker after 15 years. So if you think it's too late to benefit, think again.

You're at Risk If . . .

- You smoke cigarettes or marijuana.
- Your diet is lacking in fruits and vegetables (for their beta-carotene).
- You are exposed to asbestos or radiation at your job.

Warning Signs

- Chronic cough or hoarseness.
- Change in cough or coughing of blood.
- Pain or shortness of breath.

Diagnostic Test

- A sputum test or chest x-ray for workers in hazardous occupations.

Recommended Schedule for Diagnostic Test

- None has been specifically designated.

Best Preventive Strategies

- Don't smoke.
- Avoid asbestos.
- Eat at least a serving of fresh fruit or vegetables daily.
- Avoid chronic exposure to high levels of radon.

Esophageal Cancer

Estimated cases in 1987: 6,800; estimated deaths: 6,400.**

Cancer of the esophagus is rare, but it is very deadly for those who do contract it. The disease can spread quickly to

*All figures given are for American men.

other parts of the body via the lymph system and blood and usually responds poorly to treatment—surgery and radiation being the two most common forms. Clearly it's a cancer not to get in the first place, and refraining from both smoking and immoderate drinking appears to be the best way to do that. Men who smoke and drink have 30 times the risk of esophageal cancer of men who do neither.

You're at Risk If . . .

- You smoke.
- You drink more than moderately.
- Your diet does not include sources of adequate vitamins and minerals.

Warning Signs

- Trouble swallowing.
- Pain and spasms in the area of the esophagus following meals.
- Recurring indigestion.

Diagnostic Test

- Medical exam.

Recommended Schedule for Diagnostic Test

- As symptoms dictate.

Best Preventive Strategies

- Don't smoke.
- Limit alcohol intake.
- Eat a balanced diet.

Colorectal Cancer

Estimated cases in 1987: 70,000; estimated deaths: 29,100.

The success of President Reagan's treatment for colorectal cancer should serve as an example for all of us: Caught early, the cancer is frequently curable. Colorectal cancer is thought to be encouraged by the high-fat, low-fiber diets typical of most American men. But a history of ulcerative colitis and a family history of polyps (intestinal growths, either malignant or benign) also can increase a

man's risks. Treatment for colorectal cancer is usually surgery, which underscores the importance of early detection. The sooner intestinal or rectal tumors are discovered, the less radical the surgery required.

You're at Risk If . . .

- You eat a high-fat diet.
- You eat a low-fiber diet.
- You get less than 800 milligrams of calcium daily.
- You have a history of ulcerative colitis.
- Your family has a history of intestinal polyps.
- You are over 40 and do not have a digital rectal exam at least yearly.

Warning Signs

- Blood in the stool.
- Feelings of being bloated.
- Change in bowel habits.
- Gas pains.
- Constipation.
- Diarrhea.

Diagnostic Tests

- Digital rectal exam performed by a physician.
- Fecal blood test performed by a physician or with a do-it-yourself home test.
- Proctosigmoidoscopy—an internal viewing of the rectum and colon via rigid or flexible tubing.

Recommended Schedule for Diagnostic Tests

- A digital rectal exam annually after the age of 40.
- A fecal blood test annually after the age of 50.
- A proctosigmoidoscopy at ages 50 and 51 and at three- to five-year intervals after that.

(This schedule should begin ten years earlier if you have ulcerative colitis or if there's a history of intestinal polyps in your family.)

Best Preventive Strategies

- A low-fat, high-fiber diet.

- Adequate intake of calcium (at least the RDA of 800 milligrams).
- Adhering to the recommended schedule for diagnostic testing.

Prostate Cancer

Estimated cases in 1987: 96,000; estimated deaths: 27,000.

Only about 2 percent of cases of prostate cancer occur in men younger than 50, but rates of occurrence are quite hefty after that—the disease is responsible for roughly 18 percent of all male cancers. Cure rates are encouraging, however, pushing 80 percent if the disease is caught early. Treatment is usually radiation, hormones, or surgery. And though impotence may be a side effect of treatment in some cases, risks have been reduced substantially in recent years. The best way to avoid prostate cancer, studies suggest, seems to be reducing fat in the diet. High exposures to cadmium (a possible problem for welders, rubber workers, electroplaters, and alkaline-battery makers) may also increase risks.

You're at Risk If . . .

- You eat a high-fat diet.
- You are exposed regularly to cadmium.
- You are over 40 and do not have regular prostate examinations.

Warning Signs

- Weak or interrupted flow of urine.
- Inability to urinate or difficulty in starting.
- Need to urinate frequently, especially at night.
- Blood in the urine.
- Urine flow that is not easily stopped.
- Painful or burning urination.
- Continuing pain in the lower back, pelvis, or upper thighs.

(These symptoms may indicate noncancerous prostate enlargement, a far less serious condition, but see your doctor to be sure.)

Diagnostic Test

- A digital rectal exam.

Recommended Schedule for Diagnostic Test

- Every year after age 50.

Best Preventive Strategies

- Avoidance of a high-fat diet.
- Avoidance of cadmium.
- Yearly checkups after age 50.

Pancreatic Cancer

Estimated cases in 1987: 13,000; estimated deaths: 12,300.

As the figures show, cancer of the pancreas is one of the most deadly forms of cancer, killing about 95 percent of the men who contract it. The problem with pancreatic cancer is that it's difficult to diagnose. Tumors usually are inoperable by the time they're discovered—which highlights the need for prevention. Research shows that men between the ages of 50 and 70 are at the greatest risk for pancreatic cancer and that smoking and a high-fat diet appear to be the major instigators of the disease. Alcoholism, diabetes, pancreatitis, working in the dry-cleaning business, and chronic, long-term exposure to gasoline also appear to increase risks.

You're at Risk If . . .

- You smoke.
- You eat a high-fat diet.
- You do *not* eat fruits and vegetables.
- You're a heavy drinker.

Warning Signs

- Jaundice (yellowing of the skin and whites of the eyes).
- Abdominal pain.
- Weight loss.
- Poor appetite.

Diagnostic Test

- Medical exam.

Recommended Schedule for Diagnostic Test

- As symptoms dictate.

Best Preventive Strategies

- Don't smoke.
- Reduce dietary fat.
- Limit alcohol consumption.
- Increase intake of fruits and vegetables.
- Pay attention to warning signs.

Stomach Cancer

Estimated cases in 1987: 15,000; estimated deaths: 8,300.

Stomach cancer is one of the few types that have declined sharply: Barely one-fourth as many cases occur today as 50 years ago. Also encouraging is the cure rate for stomach cancer if it's diagnosed in time—roughly 75 percent. If diagnosed in late stages, however, the five-year survival rate drops to 10 percent. Major risk factors for the disease include smoking and a diet rich in smoked, salted, pickled, or high-nitrite foods. Surgery is usually the most successful treatment, and a diet rich in fruits and vegetables is thought to protect against the disease.

You're at Risk If . . .

- Your diet is rich in smoked, salted, pickled, or high-nitrite foods.
- You rarely eat fruits and vegetables.
- You smoke.
- You have pernicious anemia.

Warning Signs

- Nausea.
- Gas.
- Burning pain after meals.
- Sensations of fullness.
- Loss of appetite.

Diagnostic Test

- Medical exam.

Recommended Schedule for Diagnostic Test

- As symptoms dictate.

Best Preventive Strategies

- Abstain from smoked, salted, and pickled foods (such as processed meats, bacon, sausage, and hot dogs).
- Eat plenty of fruits and vegetables.
- Don't smoke.

Bladder Cancer

Estimated cases in 1987: 33,000; estimated deaths: 7,200.

Slow to spread and highly curable, bladder cancer nonetheless manages to kill more than 7,000 men every year. The cancer occurs mostly in white men over the age of 65 and also tends to occur in people with a history of bladder infections. Chemotherapy, radiation, and surgery are the most common forms of treatment. Survival rates, if the disease is discovered early, average about 70 percent. Again, smoking appears to be the greatest risk factor for bladder cancer. House painters, truck drivers, textile workers, chemical workers, metal workers, machinists, and printers also may have slightly elevated risks.

You're at Risk If . . .

- You smoke.
- You have a history of bladder infections (and do not get treatment promptly).
- You work in an increased-risk profession.
- You're 65 or older.

Warning Sign

- Blood in the urine.

Diagnostic Test

- Medical exam.

Recommended Schedule for Diagnostic Test

- As symptoms dictate.

Best Preventive Strategies

- Don't smoke.
- Seek medical attention promptly for bladder infections.
- Seek medical attention promptly for blood in the urine (which can be caused by other, less serious conditions, but it's best to play it safe).

Oral Cancer

Estimated cases in 1987: 20,200; estimated deaths: 6,350.

Oral cancers include those of the tongue, the floor of the mouth, the soft palate, the tonsils, the pharynx, the lips, the insides of the cheeks, and the gums—and 70 percent occur in men over 45. Tobacco—either smoked or chewed—appears to be the greatest risk factor, but there is evidence that alcohol increases risks as well. Combine the two and you've got double trouble: Studies suggest that men who both smoke and drink may boost their risks by as much as 15 times. Deficiencies in vitamin A and the B-complex vitamins also can elevate risks, as can irritations or infections of the mouth.

You're at Risk If . . .

- You smoke or chew tobacco.
- You drink alcohol.
- You are deficient in the B-complex vitamins or vitamin A.
- You have dental problems that cause irritation or infection.

Warning Signs

- White, smooth, or scaly spots on the lips or in the mouth.
- Swelling or lumps in the mouth or on the neck, lips, or tongue.
- Numbness, burning, dryness, or pain for no known reason.
- A sore or red spot that doesn't heal in two or three weeks.
- Repeated bleeding in the mouth with no known cause.
- Trouble speaking or swallowing.

Diagnostic Test

- A self-exam or an exam by your dentist.

Recommended Schedule for Diagnostic Test

- As often as you see your dentist, which should be every six months.

Best Preventive Strategies

- Don't smoke or chew tobacco.
- Limit alcohol intake.
- Get adequate levels of B-complex vitamins and vitamin A.
- Seek treatment promptly for dental problems that cause mouth, lip, or tongue infections or irritations.
- Seek treatment for the development of any of the abnormalities of the mouth mentioned above.

Liver Cancer

Estimated cases in 1987: 7,100; estimated deaths: 5,300.

The liver is an amazingly regenerative organ, capable of returning to its original size and health even after being reduced by as much as 80 percent by surgery. A cancerous liver, however, is not capable of such miraculous regrowth, which is why most liver cancers prove fatal. Fortunately, liver cancer accounts for only 1 or 2 percent of all malignancies. The greatest risk factors appear to be cirrhosis, which is often caused by heavy drinking; hepatitis, which strikes hemophiliacs and intravenous-drug users; poor nutrition; and occupational exposure to vinyl chloride.

You're at Risk If . . .

- You're a heavy drinker.
- You've ever had hepatitis or cirrhosis.
- You're exposed to vinyl chloride at your job.
- You are poorly nourished.

Warning Signs

- Loss of appetite.
- Weight loss.

- Abdominal swelling.
- Malaise, fever, jaundice, or pain.

Best Preventive Strategies

- Abstain from intravenous drugs.
- If you are a hemophiliac, have regular checkups for exposure to hepatitis.
- Moderate drinking.
- If you are exposed to vinyl chloride on the job, have regular medical checkups.
- Eat a nutritious diet.

Skin Cancer

Estimated cases in 1987: 13,600; estimated deaths: 4,800.

The major cause of skin cancer is the sun, and the major skin cancer sites are those parts of the body the sun hits most: the face, the backs of the hands, the tops of the ears, and yes—in bald men—the top of the head. Skin type also determines susceptibility: The fairer the skin, the greater the risk. Skin cancer is the most common form of cancer, but it's also the most curable. Only melanoma has the potential for being fatal, but even melanomas are highly curable if caught in time (see warning signs below). In addition to sunlight, certain drugs used to treat psoriasis (crude-tar ointments and chemicals called psoralens) can increase skin cancer risks. So can occupational exposure to coal tars, pitch, asphalt, soot, creosotes, and lubricating and cutting oils.

You're at Risk If . . .

- You have fair skin.
- You enjoy pursuing a dark tan.
- You have an outdoor job or spend lots of leisure time outside.
- You're being treated with crude-tar ointments or psoralens for psoriasis.
- You're exposed to coal tars, pitch, asphalt, soot, creosotes, or lubricating and cutting oils on the job.
- You've had more than an average number of x-rays.

Warning Signs

- A sore that doesn't heal in six weeks.
- Lumps or growths that keep bleeding or enlarge, especially if they're firm to the touch.
- Any mole that looks splotchy, brown, or black or has an uneven border (like a maple leaf).
- A mole or other growth that changes size or shape.
- A mole that itches or feels sensitive.

Diagnostic Test

- Self-exams.

Recommended Schedule for Diagnostic Test

- At least once annually.

Best Preventive Strategies

- Avoid direct sunlight between 10:00 A.M. and 2:00 P.M. (11:00 A.M. and 3:00 P.M. during daylight saving time).
- Use a sunscreen with an SPF (sun protection factor) of at least 15 if you must be in the sun, and reapply every 2 hours.
- Wear protective clothing, including a hat, when in the sun.
- Check with your doctor to see if any medication you are taking increases your sensitivity.
- Avoid tanning salons and sunlamps.
- Remember that reflective surfaces like snow, water, cement, and sand can reflect burning sun rays onto your skin, even if you're sitting in the shade.

PART V: BETTER WAYS TO BEAT EVERYDAY HEALTH PROBLEMS

CHAPTER 19
How to Tell Your Doctor What Hurts

Accurately communicating your problem is the key to a proper diagnosis.

You have decided to see a physician either because you have symptoms or want a checkup. You have received the name of a doctor from family or friends. You have called and made an appointment. You have, it is hoped, even found out what kind of physician he or she is. Is that all you need do?

No! Now you have to prepare to succeed where many, many patients fail: You have to tell your doctor what is wrong with you.

The first several minutes of contact between you and your physician are going to be spent on your medical history, the details of the current symptoms, and the recitation of your past medical problems. Despite the proliferation of blood tests, scans, and other diagnostic tools, the medical history is still by far the most important factor in the making of a diagnosis.

You should be able to present a fairly precise story and be able to answer your doctor's questions. Do not begin with broad generalizations or gross exaggerations, such as "I don't feel good," or "Everything hurts," and then lapse into silence.

The time to begin the process of analyzing your complaints is *not* while you're sitting in the doctor's office. So before you go, while you still have time, learn something about symptoms.

Body and Pain Specifics

Pain is probably the most common symptom. Know when the pain began, as precisely as you can determine. Know if the pain is the same as when it began or if it is getting worse. Pay attention to whether the pain travels or radiates, and whether it is constant or intermittent. If it is intermittent, how long do you feel it? How long does it stay away?

Be specific with the part of the body you identify. A woman once complained to a doctor about her "arthritis" pain and said that she had not experienced relief from the arthritis pills prescribed by another doctor. When asked where her pain was, she stated that it was in the knee, pointing then to a spot on her leg several inches below the knee. The woman had superficial phlebitis—not arthritic pain at all. Certainly the physician she saw first should have made the proper diagnosis. But who's to say what would have happened if she had told the physician that her *leg* hurt?

Abdominal pain. Do not confuse the words *stomach* and *abdomen.* The stomach is a pouch in the upper abdomen, in the soft area between your ribs. It is part of the gastrointestinal tract and receives swallowed food. The abdomen is the front of your body from the lower border of your ribs to the pelvis.

If you have or had pain in the abdomen, where in the abdomen exactly? Is it above or below your belly button? Is it central, or left or right? Does it go or radiate anywhere, up or down, left or right, into the chest or back or groin? If it does go to the back, does it go "around" your body to the

back or "through" your body to the back? Where exactly do you feel it? A variance of just a few inches can be indicative of different conditions.

When did the pain really begin? Often patients state that a pain began a week or so ago, and later the doctor finds out that it really began a year ago, lasts a week or two, and then goes away for a while.

Is it a constant pain, or does it vary in intensity? Does the time of day matter? Is it related in any way to your menstrual cycle? Does the position of your body matter? Is the area that hurts tender? (Tenderness means that it hurts more when you touch it.)

Does eating have any effect on your pain? Does it make it better or worse? If eating has an effect, when does it happen—as soon as you start eating, a few minutes later, or an hour later? Again, if eating affects the pain, does it matter what you eat?

Does moving your bowels or urinating affect the pain, or does the pain make you want to do either of those? Does sexual intercourse affect the pain? When the pain is at its worst, do you want to lie still, or do you move around a lot (squirm)?

Are there any associated symptoms with the pain, such as fever, sweating, nausea, vomiting, belching, heartburn, shortness of breath, or flatulence (passing gas)? To a physician these specifics are not just very important; they are *crucial*!

Chest pain. A doctor will want to know a lot of specifics about chest pain. Where is it exactly? Does it radiate or go anywhere, such as your neck, jaw, teeth, back, abdomen, shoulder, or arm? What kind of pain is it? Is it sticking, stabbing, burning, pressing, squeezing? Does regular breathing make it worse? Does deep breathing or coughing make it worse? Have you been coughing? Does the movement of your body affect the pain? If you move or swing your arms, is it worse? Is the area tender, does it hurt more if you touch it? If you are not sure, press on it!

Arm or leg pain. If you have pain in an arm or leg, where exactly is it? Is it in a joint? Is the area tender to the touch? Has it ever been red or swollen as compared to the other limb? Does lying, sitting, standing, or walking affect

it? If it happens when you walk, how far do you walk before you feel it? Will the pain go away if you stand still? If you sit? If you lie down?

If the pain is in a joint or joints, which joints? If it is in a hand or finger, which joints and which fingers? Know which fingers specifically bother you; certain conditions affect some fingers and not others. Look at your fingers and notice that each has *two* joints. Different kinds of arthritis affect different joints, so know which specific joints hurt.

Back pain. If it is your back that is bothering you, where exactly does it hurt, and since when? If you point to a spot just 2 or 3 inches from where you actually felt or feel it, you are going to mislead your doctor. Does breathing, coughing, eating, urinating, or moving your bowels affect it? Does the pain go anywhere, around to the front, to your groin, into a buttock, down a leg? Which part of the leg? Does the position of your body make a difference? What time of day is it the worst? How does it feel in the morning? Did you lift or move something heavy?

Key Questions and Answers

Constitutional symptoms refer to the general condition of your health.

Has your appetite been affected? Your thirst? If your doctor asks you, "How's your appetite?" do not start telling him or her what you eat! Appetite is the "desire" to eat. And it does not help to say that you have never been a big eater. The doctor wants to know if there has been a *change.*

If you have lost your appetite, has there been any nausea? What happens if you do eat? What do you feel? Have you lost any weight? Again, be as specific as possible. Weigh yourself before you go for your checkup if you are not sure. Notice if your clothes are looser. Try to know how much weight you have lost and when the weight loss began.

Have you had any fever, chills, or sweating? Take your temperature if you feel warm. Take it an hour or so after a chill. Are you sweating more than normal—more than can be accounted for by the air temperature and your

activity? The usual sequence is chills, then fever, then sweating.

Are you more tired than normal? Are you more tired than you were a year ago? Do you become fatigued more easily upon exertion?

If you are coughing, are you bringing up any phlegm? If so, what color? Look at it! If you have phlegm, are you coughing it up from your lungs or just clearing your throat? The phrase *spitting up* is especially vague. Patients use it to describe vomiting, coughing up something from the lungs, and clearing the throat.

Do you have any pain, burning, or discomfort when urinating? If you do, mention it even if it is minimal. And pay attention to the following: When did it begin? Did it ever happen before? If you're a man, is there any discharge from the penis; if you're a woman, is there discharge from the vagina? Any stains in your underwear? How often do you have to urinate during the day, and how often during the night? Count the number of times and write it down! Do you have to go in a hurry, or can you hold it in?

Pay attention to the force of the urinary stream. Is it a strong, steady flow or does it dribble or trickle? How much urine comes out each time? Are you just urinating smaller amounts more frequently or passing a greater quantity of urine? Look at the color of the urine. Any change? Any discomfort associated with sex?

Has there been any change in your bowel habits? Do you go less often or more often? How often? Has there been any change in the color or the consistency of the stool? Is there pain or discomfort associated with moving your bowels? Where? Do you see any mucus or blood?

Have you been experiencing shortness of breath (dyspnea)? This is a very common complaint and has many different causes. Before you see a doctor, take five minutes to learn more about your particular shortness of breath. Are you really feeling a shortness of breath or are you experiencing a feeling of weakness or a feeling of heaviness or tightness in the chest? Is your breathing heavy? Are you panting? When does this shortness of breath occur? Does it happen only with exertion, such as walking, and if so, after how far? Ten steps? Ten blocks? Or does it happen

even if you are resting or sitting? How long does it last? Is there any pain, palpitations, dizziness, or other discomfort associated with it? How long ago did your shortness of breath begin? A week? A month? Five years? Is it getting worse, or is it more or less the same as when it started?

Do you suffer from dizzy spells? Again, you have to pay attention to the specifics. What exactly do you mean by dizzy? Do you feel as if you are going to faint or black out? Is it a sense of loss of balance that you feel? Is it constant or intermittent, and if the latter, when exactly does it occur? Does it happen only when you stand up from a lying or sitting position, or when you move your head regardless of the position of your body? Patients often say they get dizzy when they bend over, but further questioning reveals they are unsure if it happens when they bend over or when they straighten up.

Previsit Checklist

There are other things you should do before your visit to the doctor's office. First, write down the specifics of everything of significance that is bothering you. If you come up with an excessively long list, however, you may overload your doctor. If there is nothing really new bothering you (all your complaints are rather chronic), and you are basically going for a checkup, tell your doctor everything. If, however, you have a new symptom or complaint that prompted you to make the visit, concentrate on that. Also write down your history, including any major illnesses, hospitalizations, and surgery.

Either write a list of all your medications and dosage strengths (which are on the labels), or bring along all of your bottles. One patient who was taking an anticoagulant developed a severe pain in his elbow and went directly to an orthopedist, neglecting to tell him about the medication he was taking. The orthopedist diagnosed arthritis and prescribed medication. After several more days of severe pain, the patient went to another physician. He was hemorrhaging into the joint. The orthopedist should have made the right diagnosis, but it's possible that the patient

could have improved the outcome had he mentioned the potent medication he was taking.

As a general rule, do not eat before going to a doctor, although drinking water is all right. The doctor may want to do blood tests, especially if it is your first visit or you have not seen him or her in a while. The normal values of some blood tests are based upon a fasting condition. That is especially true for measurements of sugar, cholesterol, and triglycerides. If you are unsure about when you can eat, call the doctor's office and ask what you should do.

Be able to provide a urine specimen. Many times patients have just urinated, so they have to drink water and wait, or come back a second time.

It is fine to take a shower or a bath before a visit, but do not douche, especially if you have a vaginal problem. You may be washing away what your doctor needs to make a diagnosis.

Do not cover a rash with medication so it cannot be seen.

Some doctors recommend that you take all your regular medications before your appointment. If continuing medication is necessary, the doctor will want to see you with the full effects of what has been prescribed.

CHAPTER 20

Shoot Down the Flu

Influenza can be a serious infection, especially if it moves into the lungs and causes pneumonia. Here's your survival course.

You're relaxing at home, feeling fine. Suddenly you develop a headache. On your way to the medicine cabinet you feel a little achy, but it's been a long day, so it's probably nothing.

Moments later, you suddenly feel terrible. You're burning up. You take your temperature: 102°F. You crawl into bed, where you remain feverish and weak for four days. You have no appetite and barely enough strength to go to the bathroom. Your cough, nasal congestion, runny nose, and sore throat make you think it's a cold, but this feels much worse than a cold. It must be the flu.

Like the common cold, influenza, or flu, is a viral infection of the nose and throat. When it strikes, most people treat it like a bad cold. But influenza is much more severe. The combination of flu and its most serious complication, pneumonia, is our fifth leading cause of death, claiming more than 50,000 lives each year—and periodically many more.

Fortunately, the most deadly type of flu can usually be prevented with a vaccine available every autumn, or treated effectively with a safe prescription drug. Alternative therapies are also available.

Pandemics

"Most people, including most physicians, don't take influenza seriously enough," says Karl Kappus, Ph.D., an epidemiologist with the Influenza Branch of the Centers for Disease Control (CDC) in Atlanta. "Flu isn't new or mysterious. Compared to AIDS or Legionnaire's disease, it's not 'news.' Most people recover uneventfully within a few weeks. But for the millions of Americans at risk for flu complications—those over 65 and anyone with a chronic illness—influenza is potentially deadly."

Some flus may also prove rapidly fatal to healthy people of all ages. "Several times each century, a supervirulent influenza virus appears, and instead of the local epidemics we usually experience each winter, there's a 'pandemic,' a worldwide epidemic," says flu expert Robert G. Webster, Ph.D., a virologist at St. Jude Children's Hospital in Memphis. "Some pandemics have killed millions."

The worst pandemic of this century, the Spanish flu of 1918–19, infected half the world's population and killed 20 million people—65,000 in the United States. An estimated 80 percent of U.S. Army deaths during World War I were

caused not by enemy fire but by Spanish flu. In fact, many historians say this flu cost Germany the war. The German army was so decimated by the disease, it could barely fight.

Medical historians believe there have been pandemics every 30 to 50 years since the dawn of history. Hippocrates wrote of a disease with classic flu symptoms that swept the Mediterranean area in 412 B.C. Flu epidemics can strike like lightning, and during the Middle Ages physicians believed the disease was "a blast from the heavens." Our term "influenza" comes from *influentia coeli,* Italian for "celestial influence." The 1957 Asian flu infected 40 million Americans and contributed to 70,000 deaths. During the Hong Kong flu of 1968–69, more than 55,000 Americans died.

Epidemiologists agree that another killer pandemic is simply a matter of time. That's why the CDC Influenza Branch continually monitors outbreaks around the world and develops a new vaccine each year against the most active flu viruses. CDC epidemiologists track the flu not only in humans but in all the species the disease infects: pigs, horses, seals, and birds. A few years ago, an influenza virus similar to the 1918 flu was discovered in turkeys in Pennsylvania. Public health officials ordered farmers to destroy 17 million infected birds.

"There's no way to know when the next killer flu will strike," Dr. Webster says, "but with growing populations of children and the elderly, we have more people at greater risk for flu-related pneumonia, whether or not we have a pandemic."

Influenza ABC's

Flu symptoms include headache, fever, body aches, sore throat, nasal congestion, runny nose, cough, and possibly diarrhea. However, symptoms vary considerably. It's often difficult to distinguish between flu and the common cold. "If an upper respiratory infection hits you like a truck, with sudden fever, weakness, and body aches, it's probably flu," Dr. Kappus says. But frequently influenza feels just like a cold.

The variability of flu symptoms is due, in part, to the three different types of influenza, designated A, B, and C. Type A flu (influenza A) is the most serious. It usually (but not always) produces sudden fever, physical collapse, and body aches. Influenza A causes many local flu outbreaks each winter and the periodic pandemics.

Influenza B may also cause sudden fever, weakness, and body aches, but the symptoms are typically less severe and don't last as long. Type B flu usually feels more like a cold. Influenza B causes local epidemics, but no pandemics.

Influenza C causes only mild, coldlike symptoms in children and adults with chronic diseases or suppressed immune systems. Type C flu is not considered a public health problem.

Influenza is a major public health problem because the infection can move deep into the lungs and cause pneumonia. Since flu-related pneumonia is potentially fatal, it's important to know if an upper respiratory infection during midwinter flu season is influenza or a cold. Unfortunately, flu symptoms vary so greatly it's often impossible to tell.

"That's why the CDC tracks influenza outbreaks so carefully," Dr. Kappus says. During the flu season, the CDC issues bulletins to health officials and the media, pinpointing outbreaks around the country. Call your physician or health department to ask about flu in your area—or anywhere you plan to travel.

Brush Fire

The common cold can be transmitted either by inhalation of virus-laden cough and sneeze droplets or by hand-to-hand contact with cold sufferers or objects they've touched, then touching one's nose or eyes. The major route of cold transmission remains controversial, but there is no controversy about flu. "Influenza spreads largely by the aerosol route," says Elliott C. Dick, Ph.D., chief of the Respiratory Virus Laboratory at the University of Wisconsin in Madison. "It spreads much more rapidly than any cold virus. Flu can spread like a brush fire. One study describes how an airline passenger with influenza A infected 72 percent of fellow travelers within 4 hours."

Like people with a common cold, those infected with flu release ("shed") virus for a day or two before symptoms develop, and continue to shed for several days after the fever has subsided. Children may shed virus for up to two weeks.

"You don't even have to get sick to spread it," Dr. Kappus says. "Many people who get infected show no symptoms, or only cold symptoms, but they can still spread the virus to others who might get really sick."

Prevention

The CDC calls annual vaccination "the single most important measure" against flu. Because flu viruses undergo frequent genetic changes, a new vaccine is developed each year.

Flu vaccine is available from physicians and public health departments, many of which provide it free to those at risk, such as nursing home residents and staff.

"Anyone can get vaccinated," Dr. Kappus says, "even pregnant women after their first trimester. But those at risk definitely should: everyone over 65, and anyone with heart disease, diabetes, asthma, or other chronic illnesses."

Flu season runs from December through April. It takes about two weeks to develop effective immunity, so authorities recommend vaccination from mid-October through November.

There are two kinds of flu vaccine, both equally effective. One is made from deactivated whole virus; the other uses only part of the virus ("split virus"). The CDC recommends the split-virus vaccine for children up to age 12 because among young people it causes fewer side effects than the whole-virus vaccine, which is recommended for everyone else.

Dr. Kappus calls flu vaccine's side effects "quite mild, especially compared to type A flu." About 25 percent of recipients experience soreness at the injection site. Five to 10 percent feel a little achy, with possibly some mild cold symptoms. Children sometimes develop a low-grade fever for a day or two. Serious reactions are virtually unheard of, except among those who are allergic to eggs, the medium

used to manufacture the vaccine. People with serious egg allergies should not be vaccinated.

Despite flu vaccine's safety, the CDC estimates that only 20 percent of Americans at risk for flu complications are vaccinated each fall. "Most people just don't see influenza as serious enough to warrant the special trip," Dr. Kappus says, "and few physicians encourage flu shots."

Physicians don't promote flu shots in part because they don't get them themselves. The CDC considers health care personnel at high risk for contracting and spreading flu, but a recent study showed that while 90 percent of health providers consider flu vaccine effective, only 24 percent of physicians and 15 percent of nurses get flu shots. Why? "A general lack of concern about influenza," Dr. Kappus says, "and fear of adverse reactions, specifically Guillain-Barré syndrome."

Guillain-Barré syndrome, a rare paralytic disorder, continues to haunt annual flu vaccination efforts a decade after it appeared as a complication of the swine flu vaccine in 1976. The swine flu bore a striking genetic resemblance to the virus that caused the killer pandemic of 1918. Worried health officials rushed to produce a vaccine, then mounted a huge campaign to get the country vaccinated, including television coverage of President Gerald Ford getting his shot. Mysteriously, the feared pandemic never materialized, but those who were vaccinated developed Guillain-Barré syndrome at ten times the expected rate. Most recovered, but several died. Flu vaccines have had a tarnished reputation ever since.

"Flu vaccine's bad reputation is completely undeserved," Dr. Kappus says. "The problems with swine flu vaccine were a fluke. Since the Guillain-Barré episode, tens of millions of people have received flu vaccine, and we've had no serious problems."

But even if everyone were vaccinated, some would still get flu, because the vaccine is only 80 percent effective. However, flu tends to be mild in those who have been vaccinated.

In addition, the flu virus can change so quickly that the vaccine might not confer immunity to the new strain. That's what happened in 1986. Midway through that year,

the CDC began developing the vaccine for that fall to prevent the two types of influenza A and one influenza B that had been active during the 1985–86 flu season. But that summer, a new type of influenza A was identified, and a supplemental vaccine had to be produced, necessitating two shots instead of just one.

Even if you don't get a flu shot, type A flu can often be prevented with the prescription drug Symmetrel (amantadine hydrochloride). Dr. Webster says Symmetrel is 65 to 85 percent effective in preventing influenza A among unvaccinated people. The preventive regimen involves taking the drug daily for 6 to 12 weeks. For people age 10 to 64 (and not suffering kidney disease), the CDC recommends 100 milligrams twice a day. Those over 65 take 100 milligrams once a day. For children under 10, consult your physician.

"Symmetrel has mild side effects," Dr. Webster says. "Five to 10 percent experience some insomnia, lightheadedness, irritability, or difficulty concentrating. But these side effects are trivial compared to a full-blown case of type A flu."

Orthodox Treatments

In addition to preventing flu, Symmetrel can also be used to treat it. Start taking the drug as soon as possible after symptoms appear and continue taking it for 48 hours after they have disappeared. Symmetrel is effective *only* against influenza A, not against influenza B or any cold virus. Despite its proven effectiveness against influenza A, Symmetrel "is not widely accepted by physicians," according to a recent study. Doctors tend to feel fatalistic about flu. If you think you may have type A flu, ask for a Symmetrel prescription.

Penicillin and the other antibiotics are powerless against influenza viruses. But they may be prescribed for bacterial complications: sinus infection, bronchitis, or pneumonia.

General Suggestions

Orthodox medicine maintains that flu that does not respond to Symmetrel cannot be cured. Physicians treat the

illness "symptomatically," the same way they treat the common cold, alleviating discomfort until the body heals itself, usually within a week or two. They recommend that flu sufferers take the following steps.

Get bed rest. Most flu sufferers feel too weak to do much else for several days. Bed rest also helps isolate the infected from the uninfected, thus limiting transmission.

Don't smoke. Smoking irritates the respiratory tract, paralyzing the cilia, microscopic hairs in the throat that remove mucus. Impaired cilia increase the risk of complications.

Drink plenty of hot fluids. Hot fluids help soothe the throat, relieve nasal congestion, and most important, replace fluids lost as a result of fever.

Don't overmedicate yourself. When flu (or colds) strike, many people rush to the medicine cabinet for one of the multisymptom cold remedies heavily advertised on TV. But authorities recommend single-action remedies for individual symptoms instead. "Combination products," says David Sobel, M.D., "may not provide enough of the specific medication you need to treat your symptoms effectively. You also run the risk of side effects from medication for symptoms you don't have." Single-symptom drugs also cost less than the multisymptom remedies.

Timed-release pills may seem more convenient, but the medication is not released uniformly. You get too much for a while, then too little. Take shorter-acting drugs more frequently.

Symptom Relief

There are also measures you can take to relieve specific symptoms.

Headache, body aches, fever. Try cool cloths on the forehead or take standard doses of aspirin, acetaminophen (Tylenol, Datril), or ibuprofen (Advil, Nuprin). Shop for the least expensive brand. Children under 18 should *not* be given aspirin for flu (or colds or chicken pox) because of an association with Reye's syndrome, a rare but potentially fatal condition that affects the brain and liver. Children should be given acetaminophen.

Fever stimulates excess perspiration, which may cause

dehydration. Since the body is mostly water, significant fluid loss can be dangerous. For any fever, drink 8 ounces of water, juice, broth, or tea every 2 hours. Consult a physician for fevers over 101°F, fevers above 100°F that last more than two days, or any fever with rash, stiff neck, severe headache, and/or marked irritability or confusion—this might be meningitis, a potentially fatal infection of the fluid surrounding the brain and spinal column.

Sore throat. Gargle with warm salt water, suck on hard candies, and increase relative humidity. The recommended salt mixture is ½ teaspoon per 8 ounces of water. Any hard candies help, but for extra pain relief, try medicated sore throat lozenges. These contain over-the-counter (OTC) anesthetics like benzocaine. To increase relative humidity, take a hot bath or shower, inhale steam from a kettle, or use a vaporizer. Consult a physician if swallowing becomes a problem, or if you have a sore throat and fever over 101°F with no other cold symptoms—this might be strep throat.

Nasal congestion. Drink hot fluids, or try a vaporizer, hot bath, or shower. At night, elevate your head with extra pillows. If you must take something and you're not pregnant or nursing, ask your pharmacist for generic pseudoephedrine or use a single-ingredient brand (Sudafed). Decongestant nasal sprays should not be used for more than three days. They relieve congestion by contracting muscles in the nose, which constrict the swollen capillaries responsible for congestion. But over time, these muscles become too fatigued to stay contracted. They relax and you suffer "rebound congestion," which may be worse than your initial congestion. Oral decongestants don't cause rebound congestion, but they may cause insomnia and elevate blood pressure. Those with heart disease, high blood pressure (hypertension), diabetes, or a history of stroke, or those who are taking antidepressant MAO inhibitors, should not take oral decongestants.

Runny nose. Use disposable tissues or take an OTC antihistamine. Ask your pharmacist for generic chlorpheniramine or buy a single-ingredient brand (Chlor-Trimeton). Consult your physician before taking antihis-

tamines if you're pregnant or nursing, or have asthma, glaucoma; or prostate problems. Possible side effects include dry mouth and drowsiness, which is aggravated by alcohol. Because of the risk of drowsiness, don't drive or operate machinery after taking an antihistamine. Antihistamines have undisputed value against allergies, but their effectiveness against runny nose caused by colds and flu is surprisingly controversial, a fact lost on most physicians. Researchers reviewed all the studies since antihistamines were discovered in the late 1940s and found them evenly divided. Half showed effectiveness; half did not. A 1976 Food and Drug Administration (FDA) panel concluded that antihistamines are ineffective against cold and flu symptoms. Nonetheless, they are widely used.

Cough. "Productive" coughs bring up mucus; "dry" coughs do not. Try to live with productive coughs. They're the body's way of clearing excess mucus from the respiratory tract. For dry coughs, try a vaporizer, take a hot bath or shower, suck hard candies, or if you're not pregnant or nursing, use a single-ingredient OTC cough suppressant with dextromethorphan. Consult a physician immediately if a productive cough brings up brown or bloody mucus, if a dry cough lasts more than three weeks, or if any cough is accompanied by fever, shaking chills, chest pain, wheezing, or shortness of breath—possible signs of pneumonia.

Diarrhea. Rare in adults, this flu symptom is fairly common in children. The major risk is dehydration. Treatment involves clear liquids (water, apple juice, club soda, etc.) and BRAT, an acronym for bananas, rice, applesauce, and toast. For severe diarrhea, try Kaopectate, which is available at pharmacies. When adults experience fever and diarrhea, they usually call the illness "stomach flu." This is a misnomer; it's probably gastroenteritis, an intestinal viral infection. "Flu" is an upper respiratory infection.

Alternative Treatments

Advocates of vitamin C for colds also endorse it for influenza. Noted proponent Linus Pauling, Ph.D., recommends 1,000 to 2,000 milligrams a day for prevention, and up to

10,000 milligrams a day for treatment. The vitamin C controversy still rages. A dozen studies show it reduces duration of symptoms by about 30 percent. A dozen others show no effect. However, the studies showing no effect all used lower doses than Dr. Pauling recommends. Dr. Pauling insists that in order for the treatment to be effective, large doses must be taken throughout the day to the point where users begin to experience diarrhea.

Folk remedies for flu include chicken soup and hot toddies, combinations of tea, honey, lemon juice, sugar, and liquor. Hot liquids prevent dehydration and help relieve sore throat and nasal congestion. Chicken soup has been shown to speed the clearance of nasal mucus. The alcohol in a hot toddy does nothing to fight the infection, but it promotes rest.

The FDA has approved several herbs for treatment of colds and flu. Herbs for topical use in inhalants to treat cough and congestion include camphor oil, eucalyptus oil (eucalyptol), peppermint oil (menthol), and thyme oil (thymol). Herbs for internal use in teas include ephedra for congestion; eucalyptus for cough and congestion; horehound for cough; peppermint and spearmint for cough, congestion, and sore throat; and slippery elm bark for cough, fever, and sore throat. These herbs are available in several FDA-approved OTC products. Many other herbs have also been used to treat flu—cayenne, chamomile, comfrey, garlic, licorice, and yarrow, among others.

Homeopathy also claims to cure flu with Oscillococcinum, a microdose of duck heart and liver. Homeopathy is extremely controversial in the United States, but Oscillococcinum is a popular flu remedy in Europe, where this alternative therapy is more accepted. Since homeopathic drugs use microdoses, adverse effects are virtually unheard of.

Complications

Many people develop bronchitis, a lingering productive or nonproductive cough, toward the end of colds and flu. Bronchitis can strike anyone, but it's associated with allergies, asthma, smoke, chemical fumes, and dry environ-

ments, such as homes with forced-air heating. Treat bronchitis with hot liquids, humidification, dextromethorphan, cough drops, or herbal remedies.

Pneumonia, a generic term for any lung infection, is the major cause of flu-related deaths. About 85 percent of flu-related pneumonia is bacterial, according to Robert B. Couch, M.D., director of the Influenza Research Center at Baylor University in Houston. When flu progresses to pneumonia, the person often seems to be recovering normally, then develops a renewed fever (up to 105°F), with severe cough, brown or bloody sputum, and rapid labored breathing (30 to 60 breaths a minute). Treatment involves antibiotics, Symmetrel, and often hospitalization.

CHAPTER 21

Fat-Fighting Doctors Open Fire

The American Society of Bariatric Physicians gives good, better, and best tips on weight loss.

A calorie is not a calorie. Master that fundamental concept and you're well on your way to successful weight loss. No gimmicks, no pills, no potions. No kidding!

The latest scientific research indicates that calories from fat are treated very differently by your body than calories from carbohydrate or protein. And therein lies your ticket to Weight Loss, U.S.A.

"Ninety-seven percent of all fat calories are converted to body fat," says Robert E. T. Stark, M.D., president of the American Society of Bariatric Physicians (ASBP), special-

ists in treating overweight people. "On the other hand, you'd have to eat a tremendous amount of carbohydrates for any to be converted into body fat. Your body has marvelous regulatory mechanisms to take care of carbohydrates and protein." A person could eat 2,000 calories of carbohydrate in just one meal without gaining an ounce, for example. That's the amount of carbohydrate present in 4 to 5 pounds of bread, cereal, and fruit! But fat is a different story. Studies have shown that even on relatively low-calorie diets—diets consisting of only 1,500 calories per day—people can become obese if 50 percent of those calories come from fat.

The fat you eat is the fat you wear.

Unfortunately, the typical American diet is loaded with the stuff. Over 40 percent of the calories we eat each day come from fat. "The American Heart Association, the American Cancer Society, the American Diabetes Association—every nutritional authority who has ever addressed the subject of fat states that we should strive to reduce the amount of fat in our diet to below 30 percent of calories," says Dr. Stark. "That approach also happens to be the best for losing weight."

Get Off on the Right Foot

But while reducing the amount of fat in your diet is the most important step to reducing the size of your clothes, it's not the only step. You need to take real steps—putting-one-foot-in-front-of-the-other steps. Physical activity is the other crucial component of successful weight loss.

In one study, doctors looked at 300 obese people who had each lost 70 pounds and kept it off. Of all the things that the people did every day, there were only two that all 300 people had in common: They had all increased their physical activity and they had all reduced the amount of fat they were eating.

Exercise throws your metabolism into high gear so you burn calories at top speed. It also keeps you from losing your muscle, or lean tissue. Failure to preserve muscle is the serious flaw in most diets and explains why they are counterproductive. Muscle tissue burns more calories. So

Just the Fats, Ma'am

The main target in your war on fat is fats. Your mission (should you accept it) is to reduce your intake of fat to 30 percent or less of total calories. But how the heck do you know the percentage of calories from fat in a particular morsel of food?

Good: Peruse a recipe for the item in question. If it contains a fair amount of butter, margarine, oil, mayonnaise, or cream, it's probably out of bounds.

Better: Be calculating. Most labels tell you the total calories and the number of grams of fat in the enclosed food. That's all you need to calculate the percentage of calories from fat. Here's what you do. Multiply the number of grams of fat by 9 (there are 9 calories in a gram of fat). Then divide by the total number of calories. The answer is the percent of calories from fat.

Best: Check out *The % Fat Calorie Tables,* a booklet by Robert E. T. Stark, M.D. In it, he lists over 1,200 common foods, conveniently categorized into percent-fat-calorie ranges. Choose the majority of your foods in the 0 to 20 and 20 to 30 percent ranges. To obtain a copy of the booklet, send $4 to Arizona Bariatric Physicians, P.C., 444 West Osborn Road, Phoenix, AZ 85013.

the more muscle you lose, the harder it is to burn calories. Your goal, therefore, is to lose the fat and nothing but the fat.

Researchers recently studied two groups of obese women. One group reduced their intake of calories by 50 percent. The other group reduced calories by only 25 percent but also increased their level of physical activity by 25 percent. The group that only dieted lost more weight. But they also lost more lean tissue. The group that exercised didn't lose as much weight. But a greater percentage of

their weight loss was from fat loss. *They ate more food and lost more fat.*

Good . . . Better . . . Best!

Increasing physical activity. Reducing fat. Sounds simple. It's not. Not unless you know how to put those principles into practice. The following guide is designed to help you do that. It will show you "good," "better," and "best" ways to deal with situations and questions that weight-loss seekers face every day. It can help you make the decisions that make or break your weight-loss effort.

All three options will take you toward your goal. How fast you want to travel is up to you—and how you feel on any particular day. So forge ahead. Get into the thin of it.

Ways to Fight a Food Craving

Good: Switch, don't fight. "I proceed from the fundamental principle that food is not our enemy," says Dr. Stark. "It's not food, it's the fats in food. So I don't mind if people have cravings. Instead of denying the desire to eat, eat something that is okay—something low in fat."

Better: Learn to substitute other pleasures for food. Your food cravings are not a physiological need (hunger), but a psychological need (appetite). The neat thing about appetite is that it subsides after about 20 minutes, whether you empty the cookie jar or not. "Food is only one of an infinite number of pleasures we can enjoy," says Howard Flaks, M.D., ASBP public-relations chairman and board of trustees member. "When you learn to substitute other pleasures for food for 20 minutes, you overcome your unnecessary psychological cues for eating. Often just 2 minutes will do the trick."

Best: Take a walk. You can't get to your refrigerator if you're walking in the opposite direction. And the exercise will burn off fat while reducing your appetite.

Times to Begin a Weight-Loss Program

Good: At the beginning of the year or the beginning of any month.

Better: When your medical condition frightens you into it.

Best: When you're committed and ready.

Absolute worst: When you need to lose weight to fit into a dress for a wedding in three weeks. "That kind of crash dieting leads you into the 'yo-yo syndrome,' " says Peter D. Vash, M.D., vice-president of ASBP. "You lose fat and muscle, then regain only fat. Your percentage of body fat is always increasing, while your ability to burn calories is decreasing."

Times of the Day to Exercise

Good: Any time that's convenient. The easier it is, the more likely you are to do it.

Better: The same time every day. "If you get used to exercising at a particular time, it becomes part of your life," says Dr. Flaks. "You'll actually feel quite uncomfortable if you don't exercise at that time."

Best: If you are obese (more than 30 percent above your ideal body weight), exercise before you eat. Recent evidence suggests that you'll metabolize your food better. If you are overweight but not obese, exercise after your meal—you'll burn more calories that way.

Why the difference?

"Researchers believe that it's related to insulin resistance in obese people," says Dr. Vash. "When they exercise, they reduce their insulin resistance. With less insulin resistance they more effectively metabolize their food."

Close, but no cigar: When you finish everything else you have to do. If exercise is last on your list, you'll never find the time.

Rewards for Doing Well

Good: Look at your thinner profile in the mirror.

Better: Look at the results of your most recent blood tests. You should be delighted at the drop in your cholesterol and triglyceride levels caused by your low-fat way of eating. When those blood fat levels go down, your risk of heart disease goes down.

Best: Cater to your senses other than taste. If you like

music, for example, give yourself a CD player or opera tickets.

Forget it, pal: Food. Give yourself anything but.

Signs of a Doctor Qualified to Help You Manage Your Weight

Good: The doctor gives you a thorough physical exam and takes your medical history before prescribing medication, and does not rely solely on medication for weight loss.

Better: The doctor doesn't run a "mill." A qualified doctor gives you ample time during weekly follow-up visits and is accessible by phone. He or she helps you talk about psychological problems, your individual eating patterns, and how you can develop new eating behaviors.

Best: The doctor has all of the characteristics already mentioned and is of normal weight. "If the doctor (or his office staff) is overweight, that doesn't invoke much confidence in the patient," says Dr. Flaks.

Things to Do If You Go "Off the Wagon"

Good: Get in touch with your doctor.

Better: Don't feel guilty. "You'll only eat more," says Dr. Flaks.

Best: Control your loss of control. "Tell yourself that you made a mistake, but you don't have to continue making mistakes," says Dr. Stark.

"Unfortunately, people think of a diet as a sort of ritual, and if they break their routine they develop a sense of guilt and shame. This unfortunately leads to a lowering of their self-esteem and makes further dietary indiscretions more likely. This is how the 'dietary failure' syndrome, which affects so many chronic dieters, begins to undermine their weight-loss progress," says Dr. Vash. "But you don't 'break' the dieting process by having one meal. Every day is a new day. The summation of all those days makes for diet success. One meal will not make you fat."

Ways to Stay Motivated

Good: Look at an old photo of your flabbier self.

Better: Imagine yourself as the thinner person you will be if you stick to your weight-loss program.

Best: Focus on your goals, preferences, wishes, and likes rather than on "shoulds," "musts," and "ought tos." "Discipline is vastly overrated, in my opinion," says Dr. Stark. "I suggest that people think in terms of their hopes and desires, not in terms of what they must or should do to have success. The latter always create more pressure. Instead, look to the future; your hopes are much more powerful motivators."

Signs of a Good Weight-Loss Plan

Good: It doesn't promise a "free lunch." A good weight-loss program does not rely solely on artificial ingredients, such as appetite suppressants, thyroid tablets, or other concoctions. "There's no substitute for regular exercise and restricting your fat intake," says Dr. Vash.

Better: The program helps you to change not only your weight but also your eating behaviors.

Best: The plan emphasizes weight maintenance rather than just weight loss. "It's not important how fast you lose the weight," says Dr. Vash. "It is important how long you keep the weight off."

Reasons to Lose Weight

Good: You hate the way you look.

Better: You hate the way you feel. "People who are fat cannot enjoy life to the fullest because they are limited physically from doing many enjoyable things," says Dr. Vash.

Best: You want to be healthier. "People who are obese have three times the risk of high blood pressure and diabetes," says Dr. Vash. "Obesity is clearly associated with heart disease and gallbladder disease. Women who are obese have a greater risk of breast and uterine cancer. And obese men have more bowel and prostate cancer."

Perfectly awful: Someone else wants you to do it. "That's a sure prescription for failure," says Dr. Stark. "If you are dieting for any reason that is not internally motivated, you are unlikely to succeed."

Types of Exercise for Weight Loss

Good: Increase your "lifestyle activities." Use the stairs rather than the elevator, for example. Park a few blocks

away from your destination and walk the extra distance.

Better: Walking, or any other activity that's slow and steady. "It's the amount of time you spend, not the speed at which you perform, that makes exercise a calorie-burner," says Dr. Stark. Low-impact aerobics is good. So is walking on a treadmill or stair-climbing machine, riding a bike or exercycle, or using a rowing machine.

Best: Any form of exercise that you enjoy. People who succeed at weight loss exercise regularly and continue to do so for life. Do you like biking, for example? Great! "The point of aerobic exercise is to move your body through space!" says Dr. Vash.

Out of the running: Any form of exercise that's pounding, punishing, or painful.

Ways to Chart Your Progress

Good: Keep track of the change in your eating habits.

Better: Look at how your clothes fit. If they're looser, you're losing fat.

Best: Measure your waist, hips, and thighs once a week. It's an accurate record of fat loss.

On the disabled list: Weight watching. "The problem is not weight, the problem is fat," says Dr. Vash. "It's very important not to focus on the scale. Weight loss could be from fluid or lean muscle—it's deceptive."

Ways to Avoid Stimulating Your Appetite

Good: Don't keep any potato chips or other fatty snack foods in the house.

Better: Make food invisible. Store it in opaque containers. Keep it off the counters. Remove serving dishes from the table.

Best: Minimize the tension in your life. Your appetite can be stimulated by worry, frustration, anger, hostility, boredom, indecision, and guilt. Deal with your problems, don't eat them.

Foods That Curb Your Appetite

"There's no food that can curb your appetite, because appetite is largely a psychological phenomenon," says Dr. Flaks.

How to Get Started at Weight Loss

Good: Dial-a-diet. The Obesity Foundation, an ASBP-affiliated organization, operates a dial-a-tape service. You can choose to hear any one of eight prerecorded tapes. Call (303) 850-0328 between 10:00 A.M. and 5:00 P.M. Mountain Time, and ask for the 3-minute tape you wish to hear (at your expense):

Tape 1: "Eating Disorders."
Tape 2: "The Comprehensive Approach to the Treatment of Obesity."
Tape 3: "Your Health and Obesity."
Tape 4: "What Should You Weigh?"
Tape 5: "Taking Time to Become Slender."
Tape 6: "Foods and Your Weight."
Tape 7: "Nutrition and Weight Reduction."
Tape 8: "Why Is It Easy to Gain Weight?"

Better: Read a good book. Here are two reliable ones: *The Fat-to-Muscle Diet,* by Victoria Zak, Chris Carlin, R.D., and Peter D. Vash, M.D. (New York: Putnam, 1987) and *Controlling Fat for Life,* by Robert E. T. Stark, M.D. The latter is available for $12 from the Arizona Bariatric Physicians, P.C., 444 West Osborn Road, Phoenix, AZ 85013.

Best: Call the American Society of Bariatric Physicians at (303) 779-4833 or the Obesity Foundation at (303) 850-0328 for more information or referral to a weight-loss doctor in your area. Obesity is often accompanied by other serious medical conditions, so you should seek a doctor's guidance before you begin.

CHAPTER 22
Clear Your Sinuses

Follow these steps to stop the siege in your head.

"Imagine someone wrapping and stuffing your head like an Egyptian mummy. That's how it feels."

"With my last attack, the pain was so bad I thought it was my last night on earth."

"The headache is so monstrous it causes sharp pains in my eyes."

For these people, the source of all this suffering is eight tiny cavities inside the head called sinuses. We all have them. But an unfortunate 30 to 50 million of us experience the wrath of periodic sinus flare-ups, and we flock to the doctor for relief in such numbers that sinus problems are among the five most common "minor" health complaints in the country.

The symptoms of sinusitis, as these flare-ups are called, may include a stuffed-up or runny nose, thick mucus that can block the nose or drain down the back of the throat, python-strong pressure, fever, and head pain. Acute attacks may last from a day to a month. Chronic conditions, while usually not as painful, may hang on indefinitely.

Why we even have those hell-raising holes, however, is a mystery. Theories surface, then sink. One thought was that sinuses made our bodies lighter, giving us faster flight in olden days from saber-toothed tigers and other nasty neighbors. "But an experiment showed that filling these empty cavities only adds 2 percent to our total weight—hardly enough difference to have given us that competitive edge," says Bruce Jafek, M.D., professor and chairman of the Department of Otolaryngology/Head and Neck Surgery at the University of Colorado School of Medicine.

"Another suggestion is that sinuses serve as vibration chambers to make our voices louder," notes Dr. Jafek. "But when you consider that certain animals with very loud

'voices' have tiny sinuses, and other animals with tiny 'voices' have large sinuses, this theory doesn't seem very likely, either."

Whatever the reason for sinuses, we're stuck with them. And if you're susceptible, there's really no way to prevent all future assaults of sinusitis. But you *don't* have to be stuck under a sinus siege that drags on and on. Here's what you need to know for next time.

Sinuses for Sure?

Many people dub themselves sinus sufferers, when actually they've got something else that mimics a sinus problem. Knowing the difference is crucial, because treatments aren't always the same.

The allergic condition known as hay fever is an example. The nasal lining of a person with hay fever becomes inflamed, causing sinusitislike symptoms such as a runny or clogged nose. Since some of the same nerves serve the nose and sinuses, it's easy to see why someone might come up with an inaccurate self-diagnosis of sinus problems. (Sinus problems may sometimes follow on the heels of hay fever, but more on that later.) In this case, treating the allergy is essential.

True sinus trouble involves one or more of four sets of cranial cavities that compose the paranasal sinuses. You have one set, called *frontal* sinuses, in the brow area over your eyes. Inside each cheekbone are your *maxillary* sinuses. Your *sphenoid* sinuses are in the upper region, deep inside, behind your nose. And your *ethmoid* sinuses, troublemakers that are more like small bunches of grapes rather than two distinct cavities, are behind the bridge of your nose.

Tiny "tunnels" connect these cavities to your nose like subway lines. The sinuses, passageways, and nasal walls are lined with mucous membranes. A normal day's work for these structures finds air and secretions flowing easily from the sinuses, through the tunnels, and out the nose. When something interferes with this process, sinus trouble begins.

Wrenches in the Works

As we've noted, allergies can often masquerade as a sinus problem. But they can also trigger the real thing. Pollen, dust, mold, and other allergens in the environment spur your system to release a substance called histamine to do battle with the offending particles. Unfortunately, histamine causes mucous membranes to swell. This inflammation can block the sinuses' drainage holes and cause secretions to pool. "When this blockage happens, pressure builds and bacteria have a chance to set in," explains Steven Schaefer, M.D., professor of head and neck surgery in the Department of Otolaryngology at the University of Texas Health Science Center in Dallas. "*Bacterial sinusitis* shows up as head pain, facial tenderness over the affected sinus, yellow or green drainage from the nose or down the back of the throat, and sometimes fever." Contact with contaminated water when swimming or diving also gives bacteria an opportunity to set up camp in sinuses.

Throbbing head pain is the calling card of *aerosinusitis.* "An engorged mucous membrane from something such as an allergic reaction can block the opening of the sinus into the nose," Dr. Schaefer says. "This can create a painful vacuum."

Allergies may also give rise to small nodules, called polyps, in the nose, sinus, or sinus passageways. These bumps set up a similar pattern of blocked air and mucus flow, stagnant secretions, bacterial susceptibility, and ultimately, sinusitis.

Another cause of sinus trouble is a deviated septum. The big clue that your sinus agony is caused by a wayward septum would be inability to breathe through one side of your nose and pain or tenderness in the sinuses on that side of your face.

Both polyps and a deviated septum are easily corrected by surgery.

Viruses can also provoke a sinus outburst. "Remember the last time you caught a cold? Chances are the virus that nabbed you first appeared as a stuffy nose with clear, runny mucus, and then things turned ugly—yellow or green secretions, postnasal drip, a slight fever," explains

Dr. Jafek, who is also spokesperson for the American Academy of Otolaryngology/Head and Neck Surgery. "This is secondary bacterial overgrowth. It's quite a pain in the head while you have it, but it tends to get better in time on its own."

Set Yourself Free

If you'd rather shorten your next respiratory prison sentence (and perhaps lessen the odds of getting another one), here's the therapeutic equivalent of a cake and file.

- Learn the dos and don'ts of blowing your nose. "If you sound like a mating elk, you're blowing too hard," says Dr. Jafek. "Too much force creates a pressure in your nose that will push bacteria and pathogens up into your sinuses. Blow gently with both nostrils, never one at a time."
- Use decongestants for sweet relief. Over-the-counter sinus relief products can help unclog you, and unclogging will ease the pain. (Over-the-counter pain relievers can also soften your headache but won't help get rid of what's bugging you.) Follow the directions on the package carefully.
- Don't rely on nasal sprays. They do provide temporary relief, but repeated use can eventually paralyze the tiny "sweeper" hairs, or cilia, that normally give the brush-off to infection-causing dirt and bacteria.
- For the same cilia-damaging reasons, stop smoking once and for all. And avoid rooms crawling with puffers.
- Resist the urge to retreat into bed. It's probably the first place you'll want to go during a bad attack. But sinus pain is even more powerful when you're prone. Likewise, ever notice that when you bend over, your head feels like a towel being rung out? The most comfortable position, and one that encourages nasal drainage, is sitting upright and leaning slightly forward, as if you're writing a letter at your desk.
- Invest in a humidifier for your home if the air is dry. Moist nasal membranes help keep viruses and bacteria

away from your sinus cavities. Electrostatic air filters screen irritating particles and are worthwhile, too.

- Try acupressure, the oriental medical art. Here's the technique: With your thumbs or fingertips, press and massage the areas right under your eyebrows that are in line with the sinus area. Move in firm, slow circles, stop, and repeat.

If these measures don't help, and you have a fever or severe pain, you need to be seen by a physician. He or she will probably prescribe antibiotics if you have an infection, and will search for the cause of your condition.

For advanced sinusitis, new diagnostic and surgical techniques make it easier than ever to break the sinus blockade.

If you suspect that allergies are instigating your sinus problems, your doctor can test for specific things to which your system reacts. Antihistamines and other medications, or a series of immunity-building shots, might bring your allergies—and as a result, your sinus problems—to heel.

Sniff Away Stuffiness

For a natural, soothing way to cut through congestion and heal irritated nasal tissues, try inhaling warm saline solution.

"We call this nasal sinus irrigation," says Bruce Jafek, M.D. "Mix a teaspoon of salt with a pint of warm water, sniff a few drops at a time into your nose, and then gently expel it. Do this several times.

"Afterward, you can apply warm, moist compresses to the area of infection while leaning forward slightly. In about a half hour, your nose should drain like a faucet—and you'll feel a lot better."

CHAPTER 23

Save Your Life with a Smile

Some experts claim that hostility can be as hard on your heart as smoking or hypertension.

Your best friend is a real gem—mild-mannered, congenial, and considerate, or so you think. Secretly, he has a Type A personality, and it's as plain as day when he gets behind the wheel of a car. When he drives down the street, he thinks, "Okay, everybody, get the heck out of my way. Don't even *think* of cutting in front of me. And never *ever* honk your horn at me when I'm stuck in traffic."

What happens to anyone who ignores his rules of the road? Do the words "felonious assault" ring a bell? Well, it may not really be that bad, but there is some cause for concern.

According to Meyer Friedman, M.D., director of the Meyer Friedman Institute in Mount Zion Hospital and Medical Center, San Francisco, this type of behavior is typical. Dr. Friedman is the cardiologist who, along with Ray Rosenman, M.D., first studied behavior marked by impatience, aggressiveness, and hostility, labeled it Type A, and offered evidence hinting that it may hurt your heart enough to kill you. (Some experts agree that Type A behavior is as big a risk factor for your heart as smoking or high blood pressure.) Dr. Friedman points out that this crazed-driver syndrome is just one of 30 or more dead giveaways for the Type A personality (some are surprisingly subtle)—and one is all it takes to label you Type A.

Do you interrupt or hurry the speech of others? Vigorously tap your fingers or jiggle your knee? Turn every game into an intense competition? Frequently try to do more than one thing at a time, like think about three different problems at once or talk on the phone while writing

letters? If so, you're a suspected Type A, says Dr. Friedman.

And Type A's are not uncommon. Three-fourths of urban males and an increasing number of women, Dr. Friedman says, are Type A's.

But the big news is that there may yet be hope for Type A's. It has been widely assumed that it's easier to make pigs do pirouettes than to alter Type A behavior. Yet in their recent landmark study, Dr. Friedman and his colleagues present evidence that Type A's can change their ways and that the change can cut their risk of heart disease.

A Change of Heart

For the new study—known as the Recurrent Coronary Prevention Project—Dr. Friedman and his fellow scientists recruited over 1,000 Type A men and women who had had at least one heart attack. The researchers gave more than half of these people special counseling on how to alter their Type A behavior. Then they monitored all participants for 4½ years to see who suffered recurrent heart problems and who altered their Type A behavior. When the researchers finally analyzed the results, they were elated.

"There was a significant decrease in Type A behavior in the people who got counseling," Dr. Friedman says. "But more important, this group had *half* as many heart attacks as those in the other group. No other therapy—not diet, drugs, surgery, or exercise—has ever achieved such remarkable results. We had demonstrated that Type A behavior isn't just associated with heart disease, but helps cause it."

But deterring doom, Dr. Friedman says, isn't the only by-product of reversing Type A behavior. "In our study," he says, "when people modified their Type A habits, they gave themselves a fuller, more productive life. They granted themselves the freedom to listen, to play, to take pleasure in friends and family, to mature, to regain self-esteem, to give and receive love. These advantages alone make altering Type A behavior worthwhile, even in people who don't yet have heart disease."

Now Dr. Friedman and colleagues at the Meyer Friedman Institute are busy using the same counseling technique to banish Type A habits in business executives, army officers, and others. And in *Treating Type A Behavior and Your Heart,* Dr. Friedman and coauthor Diane Ulmer insist that Type A's can even apply this counseling on their own to change their ways.

Here are some tips from Dr. Friedman on how to use this method of self-counseling to get out of what may be the world's deepest behavioral rut.

Not Me, Not Me!

The first step, says Dr. Friedman, is discovering for yourself that you're really a Type A. But if you are, wouldn't that fact be perfectly obvious to you?

"Not necessarily," Dr. Friedman says. "The main exterior signs of Type A behavior are aggravation, irritation, anger, and impatience—what we abbreviate as AIAI. They're overt but still often hidden from the Type A. Generally, Type A's are great at spotting Type A behavior in others but awful at detecting it in themselves."

So if you're Type A, how can you accurately assess your own behavior? Be honest with yourself, says Dr. Friedman, and get a second opinion from your spouse or friends. Then take their comments seriously, even if you don't like what you hear.

Here are some of the questions you should ask yourself (and the people who know you).

- Do you have a compulsion to win at all costs, even in trivial contests with children?
- Do you clench your fist during ordinary conversation?
- Do you have easily aroused irritability or anger, even in minor matters?
- Do you have a ticlike grimace, in which the corners of your mouth are twitched back, partially exposing your teeth?
- Do you sigh frequently?
- Do you have trouble sitting and doing nothing?
- Do you detest waiting in lines?

- Do you eat, walk, or talk fast?
- Do you often angrily defend your unshakable opinions?
- Do you grind your teeth?
- Do you nod your head while speaking (rather than while listening, as many people do)?

"Few Type A's exhibit *all* the Type A signs," Dr. Friedman says. "But most Type A's have several. We have found that exhibiting even one of them (mild Type A) increases your risk of having a heart attack before age 65."

Axing Type A

So are you a Type A or not?

If you are and you admit you are, you're halfway to kicking Type A habits, says Dr. Friedman.

The next step is to deal with the cause of your Type A behavior. And guess what? The cause is not rush-hour traffic, your blockhead boss, or your neighbor's yappy dog. It's low self-esteem and insecurity, Dr. Friedman says.

"We observed," he says, "that every one of the 592 people who received Type A counseling in our study harbored insecurities and in most cases low self-esteem. Every single one of them doubted that he or she possessed the necessary abilities to perform present and future duties well enough to merit promotion.

"Typically, Type A's struggle to achieve more and acquire more in less time, thus bringing on all the AIAI symptoms. And this struggle is a way of compensating for these feelings of insecurity and inadequacy. Eradicating the feelings is sometimes a matter of discovering what past events triggered them, or ensuring that your expectations do not vastly exceed your capabilities, or even getting professional counseling."

Along with wrestling with the sources of your Type A behavior, you also have to change the false beliefs that feed it. Here's a hard-core Type A talking: "I don't want to be anything but Type A. Type A's make the world go round. Their aggressiveness gets things done. Their impatience kicks butts and makes things happen. Besides, I

have to expect a lot from myself to get ahead. And even if you put a gun to my head, I couldn't change one iota."

Here's the voice of realism talking back: "Since when does your tendency to become easily irritated, aggravated, and angered about innumerable things and persons help you succeed? And does your impatience really help you make timely decisions—or force you to jump the gun with half-baked bunk? If Type A's get things done, they do so in spite of their Type A behavior, not because of it. Fact is, Type A's don't run the world; plenty of Type B's (calmer, less harried people) dominate, too. And high expectations don't help you get ahead. They doom you to fail. Most important, you *can* change. So say science and hundreds of reformed Type A's."

This kind of point and counterpoint has to happen in your head, says Dr. Friedman, until you've replaced every bit of Type A nonsense with hard facts.

Drilling for Life

Now comes the hard part: the repetitive drills. These are behavioral exercises designed to root out Type A habits and replace them with healthier ones.

"Old habits die hard, as our study participants discovered," Dr. Friedman says. "It took months of doggedly executing the drills to kick the ingrained harmful habits. At first, the participants just went through the motions. Then, slowly, the repetitive actions began to change how the participants felt, until new habits seemed as natural as breathing."

There are two types of drills, says Dr. Friedman: general and specific. You do the general ones as often as possible, on no particular timetable. You do the specific drills according to schedule—a different drill once a day for seven days, then repeat the sequence week by week throughout the month. You try a different set of seven drills for each month. For best results, select specific drills from the list below and schedule them throughout a full year.

If you're a diehard Type A, these drills will drive you nuts—at least at first. On the other hand, they can't be any worse than a heart attack.

General Drills

Here are some general drills; remember to do them often.

- Announce to your spouse and friends that you intend to turn over a new leaf, to whip your AIAI.
- Start smiling at other people and laughing at yourself.
- Stop trying to think or do more than one thing at a time.
- Play to lose, at least some of the time.
- When something makes you angry, immediately make a note of it. Review the list at the end of each week and decide objectively which items truly merited your level of anger.
- Listen, really listen, to the conversation of others.

Specific Drills

Combine these drills into seven-day schedules, a different drill per day, repeating each schedule throughout a month.

- For 15 minutes, recall pleasant memories.
- Don't wear a watch.
- At the supermarket, get in the longest checkout line.
- Do absolutely nothing but listen to music for 15 minutes.
- Buy a small gift for a member of your family.
- *Cheerfully* say "Good morning" to each member of your family and to people you see at work.
- Carefully and slowly scrutinize a tree, a flower, sunset, or dawn.
- Walk, talk, and eat more slowly.
  On two different occasions, say to someone, "Maybe I'm wrong."
- Tape-record your dinnertime conversation, then play back the tape to see whether you interrupt or talk too fast.

So, how long must Type A's strive to be Type B's? Always, says Dr. Friedman. "I beg you to continue to save your life—year after year."

PART VI: WOMEN'S HEALTH NEWSFRONT

CHAPTER 24

The D and C: Make Sure You Need It

By Herbert H. Keyser, M.D.

This second most commonly performed operation is not always the best option—especially for premenopausal women.

In all of gynecology, no procedure is less understood by patients than dilatation and curettage—the ubiquitous "D and C." Though doctors at times affectionately call the procedure a "Dusting and Cleaning," a more accurate name might be "Dollars and Cents."

The D and C is a relatively simple operation. In this procedure—the second most frequently performed operation throughout the United States—the lining of the uterus is scraped off (curetted) after the opening of the uterus has been stretched (dilated).

The D and C often has great value, for it allows a physician to examine the contents and lining of the uterus with relative ease. Sound reasons for doing a D and C include postmenopausal bleeding, abnormal premenopausal

bleeding, polyps, miscarriages, and a number of less common disorders.

Government studies now indicate that almost 1 million D and C's are performed each year in this country. There is no question that many of these operations are performed for perfectly valid reasons. But it is also clear that many are performed for questionable reasons, especially in young women.

Necessary or Not?

When a women under the age of 40 develops some type of menstrual irregularity, there are several possible causes. The bleeding can be caused by fibroids, polyps, or even malignancy, but the most likely problem by far is hormonal: "dysfunctional uterine bleeding." That diagnosis refers to some abnormality in the delicate hormonal balance of the pituitary, hypothalamus, and ovaries.

In such women, the best treatment for menstrual irregularity is often doing nothing but waiting watchfully. Time and again in my practice, I have observed young women whose heavy or irregular menses corrected themselves once the stress in their lives was resolved. Sometimes just knowing that no serious physical problem existed was enough to reassure the patients, and their periods reverted to normal without further intervention.

If dysfunctional uterine bleeding persists, a doctor can rightfully conclude that some form of treatment is needed. But even then, several measures should be tried before surgery is contemplated.

Dysfunctional bleeding is the body's defective attempt to shed the lining of the uterus—the endometrium—in the course of menstruation. Years ago, surgery in the form of a D and C was the only way to remove the old uterine lining and allow the patient's natural hormones to create a fresh lining that would shed more regularly in the course of monthly flow. Today it is known that judicious use of hormonal therapy can often achieve the same result without surgery. There are legitimate instances when a D and C is needed by a young woman whose bleeding cannot be

controlled by medical means, but these occasions should be few and very far between.

What about women in their forties who are approaching menopause? Menstrual irregularities are not uncommon at this time.

If periods become more widely spaced, nothing need be done. If periods are heavier but regularly spaced, or if bleeding occurs between periods, an endometrial biopsy may be advisable. If bleeding persists between periods, a D and C may be necessary even in the face of an endometrial biopsy.

Endometrial biopsy is simpler and safer than a D and C because it does not require stretching of the cervical opening or the use of anesthesia. The usual fee for an endometrial biopsy is about $50, while physicians usually collect $350 or more for an average D and C! The two procedures are almost equally effective as a screening device to rule out the presence of underlying malignancy.

Menstrual Problems

Several other conditions can underlie repeated uterine bleeding in premenopausal women. One of these, cervical polyps, which are small and almost always benign, can cause abnormally heavy or irregular menstrual flow. These growths can easily be seen on examination of the cervix and can usually be removed in a simple office procedure.

The polyps that occur on the cervix are of two varieties, stalked or flat. If stalked polyps are small, they can be removed in an office procedure with a minimum of bleeding. Flat polyps, on the other hand, are more likely to bleed when removed. In my opinion, hospital-based surgery is advisable only when a danger of excessive bleeding exists.

A patient really has no way to evaluate whether the procedure should or should not be done in the office. Her only recourse is to request a second opinion if removal outside of the office is suggested.

Some D and C's are performed for the purpose of removing an intrauterine device (IUD). If a patient using this form of contraception experiences abnormally heavy peri-

ods, her physician may correctly elect to remove the IUD and wait several months to see if the excessive bleeding subsides. Physicians can claim that they are unable to remove the IUD in the office or that the bleeding might be caused by something other than the IUD. However, excellent instruments are available to handle most of the infrequent problems of difficult removal, and the bleeding is almost always certainly caused by the IUD.

If the IUD were removed in a hospital, the total cost would exceed $1,000. In an outpatient surgical unit, the cost would be about $100 less. Removal in a doctor's office can be done for the price of a routine office visit, usually $20 to $25!

Postmenopausal Bleeding

The onset of uterine bleeding in older women who have stopped menstruating is quite another matter. Spontaneous bleeding or spotting in a postmenopausal woman is a matter for some concern.

Many cases of postmenopausal bleeding occur in women who are taking an estrogenic hormone to relieve the symptoms associated with menopause. In such cases, the rational medical approach is to stop the hormone, get an endometrial biopsy, and observe the patient closely to see whether the bleeding stops.

Considerable research indicates that judiciously used hormones can have great value both in alleviating the symptoms of menopause and in preventing some of the conditions associated with aging in women. Although it is generally accepted that estrogenic therapy may cause a small increase in the malignancy rate, some of that increase may be caused by improper or excessive use of these hormones. Overall, the great majority of patients treated with the smallest effective dose of female hormones will not develop cancer or unpleasant side effects, and a number of advantages will result from their use.

Although malignancy is rare, postmenopausal bleeding caused by the use of hormones is fairly common. So doctors who prescribe hormonal therapy should be aware that a significant percentage of recipients will bleed. They

should also be willing to take time to explain to their patient that vaginal bleeding may occur. Physicians who are not fully aware of these side effects—or who choose to disregard the fact that their therapy can underlie unusual bleeding—may rush to perform what is usually an unnecessary D and C rather than an endometrial biopsy. Physicians of this bent try to justify the surgery as necessary to rule out cancer.

The far more rational treatment would be to stop administering the hormones for a few months. Endometrial biopsy should also be performed during this time to look for an underlying malignancy. If the bleeding stops, it is safe to infer that hormonal therapy caused the problem.

Endometrial biopsy, which obtains a small sample of the uterine lining, is not as definitive as a D and C for ruling out endometrial cancer. However, the chance that an early malignancy will be missed is extremely unlikely. If bleeding occurs after the hormones have been stopped, a D and C should definitely be performed. With only limited knowledge of the possible complications, an operation described as "simple" sounds logical to the patient, but it isn't. In the cold, impersonal terms of medicine, the overall complication rate of D and C's has been found by different surveys to be from 0.63 to 1.7 percent. These figures are only for D and C's unrelated to pregnancy; the complication rates of the procedure done following miscarriage or incomplete abortion are significantly higher.

These figures reflect only immediate or short-term complications that arise at the time of surgery or shortly thereafter.

What are the risks? First, any surgery using general anesthesia carries some risks—ranging in severity from the mild discomfort of nausea to the possibility of cardiac arrest and death. In addition, several complications are specific to the D and C.

Perforation of the wall of the uterus. This complication is not rare. The uterus is an internal organ that must be explored from an external opening. Thus the operating field is necessarily limited, and the surgeon cannot view the site of the surgery, the uterus itself. The operation is risky because the instruments used to perform the proce-

dure—cervical dilators to enlarge the opening and curettes to remove the contents—are sharp and relatively pointed. Women who subsequently undergo abdominal surgery are sometimes found to have uterine scars indicating that an unrecognized perforation had taken place. Although perforation may not cause major aftereffects, any accidental entry into the abdominal cavity is a potentially serious event. Infection, internal bleeding, and damage to the bladder and intestine can occur.

Excessive bleeding. This is another hazard of a D and C. When bleeding cannot be controlled by any other means, an emergency hysterectomy must be performed. Though rare, to a woman who has not fulfilled her reproductivity desires, this is an especially unfortunate consequence of this "minor" surgery.

Infection. This is a risk of any invasive procedure. In young women, infection can damage the fallopian tubes, which are critical for pregnancy and childbearing.

Scarring of the uterine lining. This infrequently occurring problem, known as Asherman's syndrome, is another result of repeated or overly vigorous D and C's.

Many of these complications of D and C are most critical to younger women, on whom the operation should almost never be performed in the first place!

I believe that a significant number of D and C's are performed in the costly hospital setting for conditions that can be treated in the doctor's office at far less cost and with far less risk to the patient. This belief was confirmed when I observed the sentinel effect: When the physicians in my institution knew that their subsequent records would be reviewed, the number of questionable D and C's dropped significantly. The main reason for this effect is that the small number of less-than-ethical physicians, who are responsible for the majority of the abuses, will provide better care when they know they are being watched.

Some unnecessary D and C's are the result of faulty rationalization; others may be motivated by greed or ignorance. Most important for patients to understand, however, is that like most unnecessary operations, inappropriately performed D and C's are almost never picked up by the institutional forces that are supposed to be protecting

the public. Tissue committees, hospital utilization committees, and even the possibility of lawsuits charging malpractice provide little or no defense against well-performed procedures. Pressure from an informed public is needed to change this situation.

CHAPTER 25

Battling Lupus

This hard-to-diagnose disease strikes ten times more women than men.

May called her father in a panic. She didn't care that she only had three more months of work before she received her Ph.D. in geology at the University of Montana. She was sick and frightened, and she wanted to be home with her parents. For close to a year she'd suffered recurrent fevers, extreme fatigue, aching joints, and sore throats. She'd taken several courses of antibiotics with no improvement. She was afraid she was dying.

May's father persuaded her to stay in Montana, and on a friend's advice, she sought care at a large medical center. There she was told she had lupus erythematosus, a surprisingly common and serious chronic inflammatory disease of the skin and connective tissue. Fortunately, May's condition responded quickly to medication and she was able to finish her studies. A doctor friend told her she was lucky. Until the 1960s, lupus was a mystery. People—usually women—developed painful joints and fever, and then died.

A Common Problem

Lupus isn't well known, but it's more common than multiple sclerosis, muscular dystrophy, cystic fibrosis, hemo-

philia, rheumatic fever, or leukemia. The disease is only now being discussed in the media, partly due to the efforts of lupus sufferers themselves to spread the word about this commonly misdiagnosed disease.

May suffered for 11 months before being properly diagnosed, but she was fortunate. According to one study, the average time between the onset of lupus symptoms and correct diagnosis is nearly five years. In North America, it affects nearly 1 million, with 50,000 new cases diagnosed annually. Although it can strike from age 5 to 75, it's most common among women of childbearing age. It afflicts women nearly ten times more often than men. Experts believe this gender difference is hormonal. Among men who contract lupus, there is an increased incidence of Klinefelter's syndrome, a feminizing chromosome disorder. Among women, blacks, Asians, and Native Americans are at greater risk than whites.

Carole, a librarian in her late thirties, suffered crying spells, depression, and lingering viral symptoms. Her doctor referred her to a psychiatrist. "I don't blame my general practitioner," says Carole. "Lupus is very hard to diagnose. My symptoms were crazy and my doctor thought I might be crazy, too." Like Carole, many people with lupus find that the vague, episodic nature of the disease increases the chance of being told "it's all in your head."

Wolf-Bite Rash

Lupus erythematosus (LE) was named centuries ago to describe the disease's characteristic rash that often spreads across the nose and cheeks and resembles the bite of a wolf (in Latin, *lupus*). The rash has also been called the lupus "butterfly mask." *Erythematosus* comes from the Greek word for redness.

Lupus is an autoimmune disorder, meaning that the body's defense mechanisms attack its own tissues. There are two types of lupus erythematosus—discoid lupus, a milder form that affects only the skin with a scaling, sometimes uncomfortable red rash, and systemic lupus, a more serious form that can attack the heart, lungs, kidneys,

brain, and particularly connective tissues such as joints and muscles.

There is no known cause, though researchers lean toward a combination of hereditary and environmental factors. Relatives of lupus sufferers have an increased risk. But among identical twins, when one twin suffers lupus, the other has only a 24 percent chance of contracting the disease, illustrating the importance of nongenetic factors. Many researchers believe that modern assaults on the immune system—drugs, chemicals, viruses, and high doses of ultraviolet light—may trigger the disease.

The most common explanation for lupus is that the immune system falsely identifies its own proteins as pathogens and sends out antibodies to "defend" the body. This forms antibody/antigen complexes that circulate in the bloodstream, causing irritation and swelling. Although lupus and AIDS may sound vaguely similar, the diseases are at opposite ends of immune system imbalance. AIDS involves destruction of the immune system; in lupus, the body's defenses overreact.

Although discoid lupus can sometimes be diagnosed by the appearance of the characteristic rash and by taking a thorough health history, diagnosing systemic lupus is much like solving a complex puzzle. The American Rheumatism Association says four of the following symptoms must be serially or currently present for a diagnosis of systemic lupus.

- Butterfly rash on cheeks.
- Discoid lupus (rash on face, arms, neck, and sometimes legs).
- Sun sensitivity.
- Mouth sores.
- Abnormal cells in the urine.
- Seizures or psychosis.
- Inflammation of the lining around the lungs and heart (pleuritis and pericarditis).
- Low white blood cell count, low platelet count, or hemolytic anemia.
- Presence of antibodies to DNA, presence of antibodies to the sm antigen (a specific antibody found in 50 per-

cent of lupus sufferers), presence of LE cells, or a false-positive syphilis test.

- Positive antinuclear antibody (ANA) test.

The most common lupus symptoms are joint swelling and pain, fever, skin changes, swollen glands, lack of appetite, nausea, vomiting, muscle aches, and painful, labored breathing. Two other common conditions, though not exclusive to lupus, are Sjogren's syndrome, which is characterized by dry, irritated mucosal surfaces such as the eyes and mouth, and Raynaud's disease, in which the hands and feet temporarily blanch white in response to cold or stress.

Lupus frequently damages the kidneys. The delicate filtration system becomes clogged by the antigen/antibody complexes, causing inflammation, functional impairment, and sometimes permanent scarring. Kidney inflammation (nephritis) can be present in lupus sufferers for long periods with no outward sign of serious damage. Kidney function must be monitored closely, since 50 percent of those with lupus develop nephritis. Kidney damage can result in high blood pressure, fluid and electrolyte imbalance, and sometimes death.

A kidney biopsy, performed under local anesthetic, in which a needle is guided via ultrasound into the kidneys, is often required to determine the extent of the damage. Susan, a 32-year-old neurobiology researcher who has lived with lupus for five years, says, "I thought the biopsy would be no big deal, but it was terrible." Although the procedure was painful for Susan, it showed she had considerable kidney inflammation but little scarring.

Central nervous system involvement often takes the form of seizures, amnesia, depression, and psychosis. Jennifer, who was diagnosed as having lupus at 14, painfully remembers her senior prom. "I stayed up late the night of the prom and then went to an amusement park, where I collapsed in a seizure and went into a coma. They rushed me to intensive care and gave me intravenous steroids. I responded pretty quickly, but it was a really scary experience. Fortunately, I haven't had a seizure since."

Among the environmental factors thought to contribute

to lupus are unidentified viruses, sun exposure, physical and emotional stress, and drugs such as birth control pills, sulfa, penicillin, barbiturates, procainamide (Procan, a heart medication), and hydralazine (Unipres, an antihypertensive). Drug-induced cases usually clear up when the offending medication is discontinued.

Treatment

Lupus is treatable, but the medications may cause serious side effects.

Anti-inflammatories. The first-line treatment is usually aspirin or nonsteroidal anti-inflammatory drugs such as Naprosyn or Motrin. Tylenol and other acetaminophen-based drugs are not helpful. Sometimes, rest and high doses of aspirin (up to 10 to 20 pills daily) are effective. But high doses of aspirin may cause nausea, ringing in the ears (tinnitus), stomach irritation, and gastrointestinal bleeding.

Antimalarials. For unknown reasons, drugs such as Plaquenil, Aralen, and Atabrine, developed to combat malaria, can alleviate the skin problems and sun sensitivity of lupus. Anyone taking these drugs should be evaluated by an ophthalmologist every four to six months because of potential vision problems associated with them. Possible side effects include vomiting and diarrhea.

Corticosteroids. These synthetic adrenal hormones are considered necessary and miraculous but often problematic. Steroids must be used cautiously and for as short a period as possible. Evidence is mounting that long-term steroid use causes premature coronary artery disease. Steroids are also associated with cataracts, loss of bone density, weight gain, mental problems, muscle wasting, and a characteristic rounding of the face ("moon face").

Steroids shut down the body's own adrenal hormone production. Sudden termination of steroids is dangerous. People are usually weaned off slowly to allow the body's adrenal glands to resume functioning.

Jennifer coped with her intermittent severe joint pains and stiffness with aspirin until an extreme flare-up landed her in an intensive care unit with a 105° fever. She was given high doses of the steroid Prednisone and her symp-

toms almost immediately disappeared. But the drugs worry Jennifer. "For three weeks, I looked in the mirror every day and asked, 'Is it happening?' So far I'm lucky. I haven't developed the steroid moon face yet."

Anti-cancer drugs. Drugs such as Imuran and Cytoxan are used in lupus treatment to decrease the immune system's responsiveness and the need for steroids. These drugs must be used carefully because they are toxic to bone marrow, which produces red blood cells.

Radiation. Less common than chemotherapy, radiation treatment involves administering relatively low doses to the lymph nodes to suppress the immune system. This technique is still experimental.

Plasmapheresis. This still-experimental technique filters the harmful antibody/antigen complexes from the blood plasma.

Living with Lupus

One of the main tasks of learning to live with lupus is accepting its unpredictable course. Some people can't, and they become reclusive and depressed. Others adopt Jennifer's attitude, "I just don't worry about anything that hasn't happened yet. If I did, I honestly couldn't get out of bed in the morning."

Rest is important. Frequently, lupus sufferers need to decrease their work schedules, particularly during flare-ups. Rest periods throughout the day are helpful. Some sufferers need 10 hours of sleep at night—or more. Since stress can precipitate flare-ups, relaxation techniques such as biofeedback and meditation may be helpful.

Get support. Most people find a lupus support group helpful, particularly right after diagnosis. Sharing coping strategies and frustrations can be both practical and comforting. Often these organizations offer classes for families of lupus sufferers to help them understand and support afflicted loved ones.

The following organizations offer pamphlets, newsletters, and other materials. Many have regional chapters. Send a stamped, self-addressed envelope for information.

- American Lupus Society, 2371 Madison Street, Torrance, CA 90505; (213) 373-1335.
- Lupus Foundation of America, Inc., 5430 Van Nuys Boulevard, Suite 206, Van Nuys, CA 91401; (818) 885-8787.
- SLE Foundation of America, 95 Madison Avenue, New York, NY 10016; (212) 685-4118.

Arrange for help with housework. Since the majority of lupus sufferers are women of childbearing age, help with housework and children is critical. Lupus and arthritis organizations offer labor-saving suggestions for household organizing.

Avoid sun exposure. Although photosensitivity varies, it's best for lupus sufferers to limit their exposure to ultraviolet light. Reactions can range from rashes and malaise to life-threatening flare-ups. Use sunscreen with a high sun protection factor (SPF), long-sleeved shirts, and hats and gloves if needed, and avoid outdoor activities during the intense midday sun. Some lupus sufferers are affected by the heat as well. For some, relocation to a cooler climate is necessary.

Exercise regularly. Exercise improves general health and provides a sense of well-being. Swimming is particularly good because it cools inflamed joints. If possible, consult a physical therapist for a personalized low-stress exercise program.

Avoid people with suspected or known contagious illnesses. Because of their poor resistance, many lupus sufferers avoid large groups during the cold and flu season.

Eat a low-fat, low-salt diet. It's easier on the kidneys and generally more healthful.

Avoid birth control pills. Although some women with lupus can tolerate birth control pills, they are generally not recommended because of the lupus/hormone link. Intrauterine devices (IUDs) are not recommended either, due to the increased risk of infection. Barrier methods such as the diaphragm or condoms are safest.

Consult a physician before considering pregnancy. Although there is an increased risk of miscarriage, recent research shows that most women with lupus are able to carry their babies to full term and deliver vaginally. How-

ever, cardiac and renal problems as well as certain medications may preclude pregnancy. Newborns occasionally show lupus symptoms, but these generally clear up spontaneously.

Consider avoiding immunizations. Consult your physician when traveling to countries requiring immunizations, as they can precipitate flare-ups. Sometimes a letter from your doctor satisfies immigration officials.

Wear or carry Medic-Alert information. This can be a bracelet, necklace, keychain, or card that describes your illness and need for regular medications.

Seek a caring, knowledgeable doctor. Lupus is a complex and frustrating disease. If you've been bitten by the red wolf, ask questions and become informed.

CHAPTER 26

Vaginitis Update

Experts agree that the key to stopping chronic infections is accurate diagnosis and treatment.

Most women suffer the itching, burning, pain, and discharge of vaginal infections on occasion. In fact, vaginitis is a prime reason women seek medical care. Many women suffer these infections again and again. The good news is that you can help yourself get off the vaginitis merry-go-round.

Vaginal infections are caused by a number of different microorganisms, many of which normally inhabit the healthy vagina. Nine out of ten women with vaginal infections are infected by one or more of the following organisms: *Candida albicans*, a common fungus that causes yeast infection; trichomonas, a one-celled protozoan; or a variety of bacteria, including *Gardnerella*.

Yeast Infections

At least 75 percent of all North American women suffer at least one yeast infection. Experts estimate that nearly half suffer multiple infections. Felicia Stewart, M.D., coathor of *My Body, My Health,* says she often sees women with recurrent yeast infections. "If the infection is recurrent, it's usually a yeast problem. Yeast infections are characterized by itching, caked discharge that smells like baking bread, and reddening of the labia and sometimes the upper thighs."

Candida organisms normally inhabit the healthy vagina. The vagina's slightly acid pH generally keeps these and other microorganisms from multiplying rapidly enough to cause infection. But many things change the vaginal environment, permitting the overgrowth of yeast or other organisms.

Pregnancy. Hormonal changes during pregnancy alter vaginal pH and increase carbohydrate (glycogen) production, which provides food for infectious organisms. Researchers estimate that approximately one-third of pregnant women test positive for *Candida.* Recurrent attacks of yeast are common among pregnant women and often increase as pregnancy progresses.

Menstrual periods. Some women are particularly susceptible to yeast infections after their periods.

Contraceptives. Under the influence of increased estrogen and progesterone from oral contraceptives, glycogen production increases. Studies show that oral contraceptives increase glycogen in the vagina by 50 to 80 percent. Although no cause-and-effect relationship has been demonstrated, oral contraceptives may contribute to yeast infections.

There is also some evidence that IUDs play a role in yeast infections. Researchers believe that the devices increase vaginal secretions, creating a more favorable environment for fungal growth.

Women who use contraceptive sponges are also more likely to develop yeast infections. "We're not sure why sponges increase yeast infections," says Dr. Stewart, "but we know they alter the vagina's normal ecology."

Antibiotics. *Candida* live in the healthy vagina in balance with other microorganisms, especially lactobacilli. Tetracycline, ampicillin, and other antibiotics kill the vagina's lactobacilli and allow the *Candida* to multiply. Some antibiotics, especially tetracycline, also appear to have a growth-stimulating effect on yeast organisms. Lois Addison, laboratory coordinator at the Family Practice Center Lab at North Carolina Memorial Hospital in Chapel Hill, North Carolina, advises doctors to recommend acidophilus capsules whenever they prescribe antibiotics. "We've found that women who take three to four acidophilus capsules with each antibiotic pill are less likely to develop antibiotic-induced yeast infections because they repopulate their lactobacilli."

Flagyl (metronidazole), a medication used to treat trichomonas and bacterial vaginosis (formerly called nonspecific vaginitis), has also been recently associated with yeast infection.

Diabetes. The high blood sugar caused by this disease promotes yeast infections. Women with recurrent yeast infections should have their blood sugar checked for diabetes or prediabetic conditions. Diabetic men may infect their partners from *Candida* organisms on the penis.

High-sugar diet. Dairy products, sugar, and artificial sweeteners may contribute to yeast infections. High sugar intake can change the vaginal pH and provide food for yeast organisms. "Some women," says Dr. Stewart, "drink lots of fruit juice to prevent bladder infections. But fruit juice contains so much sugar that it may promote yeast infections."

Tight clothing and personal habits. Tight, insulating clothing such as panty hose and bathing suits provide the ideal combination for yeast growth: poor ventilation and heat. Feminine hygiene sprays, deodorant toilet paper, and commercial douches may irritate vaginal tissue and predispose women to yeast infections. Although no studies confirm a tampon/yeast infection link, some women believe tampons play a role in their recurrent yeast infections. Tampons, especially the superabsorbent variety, may dry and irritate the vagina.

Yeast Treatments

Physicians generally treat yeast infections with any of three medications: Mycostatin or Nilstat (nystatin), Monistat (miconazole) or Gyne-Lotrimin (clotrimazole). The treatment course for Mycostatin or Nilstat is usually one suppository every 12 hours for one to two weeks; for Monistat and Gyne-Lotrimin, suppositories nightly for three days or cream once daily for one week. Dr. Stewart says, "In my experience, miconazole and clotrimazole are much more effective than nystatin for treating yeast." Researchers are experimenting with single-dose suppositories, but results have been mixed. Gentian violet can provide immediate relief from yeast symptoms, but because some women have severe reactions to this dye, most doctors opt for antifungal creams or suppositories.

Although there are few, if any, good studies to confirm their effectiveness, some women report success with self-care yeast remedies. You might try douching with a mild vinegar or yogurt solution at the first sign of infection. For a vinegar douche, use 1 to 3 tablespoons of vinegar to 1 quart of warm water; for a yogurt douche, make a dilute mixture of plain yogurt and warm water. Some women find relief using Lactinex (lactobacillus) tablets vaginally (one or two daily) and vinegar douches twice a day for two days. Other home remedies for yeast infections include goldenseal-myrrh douches (simmer 1 tablespoon of each in 3 cups of water for 15 minutes, strain, and cool) and garlic suppositories (peel one clove without nicking, wrap in gauze before inserting, and leave in for 12 hours).

Several studies have shown boric acid to be a safe, inexpensive, and effective remedy. Dr. Sadja Greenwood, women's health editor for *Medical Self-Care* magazine and coauthor of the *Medical Self-Care Book of Women's Health,* suggests 600-milligram boric acid capsules daily for 14 days as a douche or a vaginal suppository.

While home remedies may work for some women, Addison emphasizes the vagina's delicacy. She says, "I've seen women who have literally burned their vaginas by douching with things like Dr. Bonner's Peppermint Soap or Lysol."

Recurrent Yeast Infections

Some researchers suggest that local therapies such as antifungal suppositories or creams may eliminate only the superficial infection, leaving live fungus in deeper tissue layers to cause reinfection. Others contend that there are "reservoirs" of yeast organisms, such as the gastrointestinal tract, that reinfect the vagina, although this theory is controversial. For recurrent yeast infections, some doctors prescribe oral nystatin to decrease the amount of *Candida* in the gastrointestinal tract. Others suggest using an antifungal cream around the anus and between the anus and the vagina to eliminate any spread to the vagina.

Male sex partners may also be a common source of reinfection. Although men rarely show symptoms, they may harbor yeast organisms, especially in the foreskin of an uncircumcised penis. In new research recently published in *Obstetrics and Gynecology,* doctors cultured the semen of the sexual partners of women with recurrent yeast infections. They found that most semen samples contained yeast organisms, probably due to prostate infection. This source of reinfection cannot be detected by simply examining the penis. The infected women were treated with a variety of standard yeast treatments and their partners were treated with 200 milligrams of oral ketocanazole for two weeks. Thirty-one of the 33 women studied remained infection free after one year. Dr. Stewart says she's had similar success treating male partners. Although the role of male sex partners in yeast recurrence needs further study, women with recurrent infections should have their partners wash extra carefully, use an antifungal cream on their genitals, and have their semen cultured for yeast organisms.

A recent study conducted by an Australian gynecologist suggests that Depo-Provera, a contraceptive administered periodically by injection, may inhibit yeast recurrence. Researchers followed 15 women on Depo-Provera, 3 of whom were given the drug specifically to control *Candida,* and found that none developed yeast infections. Two longtime sufferers of recurrent *Candida* infections reported their first relief in several years from the Depo-Provera treatment. Side effects of this drug may include breast tender-

ness, increase or decrease in weight, edema, insomnia, nervousness, depression, fatigue, dizziness, headaches, skin problems such as acne, and hair growth.

Other suggestions for treating recurrent vaginal infections include:

- Using prescribed medication for a longer period of time, even during menstruation. Ask your doctor for an open prescription for vaginal cream or suppositories.
- Using an antifungal cream or suppository for a few days before your period and/or a few days after.
- Using vaginal antifungal medications during and for several days after taking antibiotics.
- Discontinuing oral contraceptives.
- Applying antifungal cream to your vulva and your partner's genitals twice daily for ten days.

Trichomonas

Approximately 25 percent of women complaining of vaginitis symptoms are infected with trichomonas, or "trick," as it is commonly called. This sexually transmitted vaginitis is caused by trichomonads, one-celled protozoans with distinctive whiplike tails, that do not normally inhabit the body. Trichomonas is characterized by foul-smelling, yellowish, frothy discharge. If the infection has extended into the urinary bladder, symptoms may include the need to urinate frequently.

Trichomonas is easily identified under the microscope. Sometime trichomonads may also be spotted during a Pap smear or in a urine sample.

Trichomonas grows best in an alkaline environment, and some women notice these infections are more prevalent after menstruation due to the alkaline nature of menstrual flow. Vinegar douches, which acidify the vagina, may be effective in reducing symptoms, especially in mild cases. Some women have had success using a douche of 4 tablespoons of vinegar and 1 to 2 *drops* of baby shampoo in 1 quart of warm water daily for one week. The trichomonads are damaged by the acidity of the vinegar and their cell walls are disrupted by the detergent in the shampoo.

The current treatment for trichomonas infections is Flagyl (metronidazole). Since the disease is sexually transmitted, both the woman and her lover must be treated. Condoms should be used during treatment. Flagyl is prescribed in 250-milligram doses three times a day for seven days, or in two 1,000-milligram doses 4 to 6 hours apart, or in a single 2,000-milligram dose.

Anyone taking Flagyl *should not drink alcohol.* Alcohol and Flagyl can cause nausea, flushing, abdominal cramps, and headaches. Other side effects of the drug may include diarrhea, dry mouth, convulsive seizures, numbness of the arms and legs, metallic taste in the mouth, and depression of white blood cell production. Some evidence suggests the shorter exposure of the single-dose treatment reduces side effects, including Flagyl-induced yeast infections.

Paul Wolner-Hanssen, M.D., an assistant professor of obstetrics and gynecology at the University of Washington in Seattle, says he's had good success with the single 2,000-milligram dose. "Most cases of trichomonas," he says, "are cured with one dose of Flagyl. In a few resistant cases, we use a higher dose and longer treatment." Although it hasn't been studied, Dr. Wolner-Hanssen says trichomonas has been successfully treated using Flagyl intravaginally without the side effects of oral administration. "It's been effective here in our STD clinic," he says, "but it needs more study. It may offer an answer to the possible unpleasant side effects of Flagyl."

Although Flagyl is currently the most effective treatment for tenacious trichomonas, several studies with laboratory mice have associated the drug with increased rates of cancer. The drug should not be used by women who are pregnant or nursing, or those with neurological disorders. Women wishing to avoid Flagyl can use the self-care vinegar/detergent douche or an antifungal cream such as Monistat (miconazole) or Gyne-Lotrimin (clotrimazole) nightly for one week.

Recurrent trichomonas is usually caused by reinfection from untreated sexual partners. Less than 20 percent of men with trichomonas are symptomatic. *All* sexual partners must be treated to avoid reinfection. Dr. Wolner-Hanssen advises, "Use condoms to protect yourself, espe-

cially with new sexual partners." Although trichomonas is usually sexually transmitted, the organism can survive in tapwater, soap, bubble baths, chlorinated swimming pools, and hot tubs. If trichomonas recurs, women should check for these sources of reinfection.

Bacterial Vaginosis

Vaginitis not caused by yeast or trichomonas is called bacterial vaginosis (BV, formerly nonspecific vaginitis). It is often caused by several bacteria, including *Gardnerella*. BV is the second most common vaginal disease in North America. The chief symptom is a foul or fishy-smelling, gray or yellowish vaginal discharge. Some women also suffer itching, low back pain, pain on urination, cramps, or irritation during intercourse. BV is easy to transmit sexually, but it may also arise spontaneously.

Researchers have found that women with IUDs are more likely to develop bacterial infections. The IUD string may act as a ladder for bacteria to enter the vagina.

BV is often overdiagnosed. According to Dr. Stewart, "BV is a 'basket diagnosis.' If some doctors can't see yeast or trichomonas, they assume it's bacterial vaginosis." She says women often see a discharge and go to the doctor complaining of vaginitis. "The doctor gives them medication, but they don't have BV symptoms, just normal discharge." Stewart says for accurate BV diagnosis there must be altered pH, abnormal discharge with characteristic BV "clue" cells present, and a foul, fishy odor.

Antibacterial douches such as Betadine (povidone-iodine) are often effective. If not, bacterial vaginosis can be treated with Flagyl, usually 500 milligrams orally twice a day for seven days. Recently, Norwegian researchers have had success prescribing 2,000 milligrams of Flagyl orally on days one and three, but other studies have shown these high doses to be less effective. Some doctors treat bacterial vaginosis with oral ampicillin or a sulfa cream. Some evidence suggests that ampicillin may be more effective than Flagyl for treating men. Cephradine, 500 milligrams four times a day for seven days, may be used for stubborn cases. Nightly douching with a 3 percent solution of hydrogen

peroxide diluted with four parts water for one week may also help. During the treatment period, condoms should be used for intercourse.

BV reinfection is common. Partners often reinfect one another in Ping-Pong fashion. Dr. Wolner-Hanssen says the role of male sex partners in recurrent BV isn't clearly understood yet, but may be a key to reinfection. "We consider an uncircumcised partner a risk factor," he says, "because women with uncircumcised partners appear to have more BV. There's also some evidence that males may harbor these anaerobic organisms in prostate fluid." The use of condoms and treating male sex partners help prevent reinfection.

Atrophic Vaginitis

After menopause, decreased estrogen production and subsequent thinning of the vaginal walls can result in a form of noninfectious chronic vaginitis called atrophic vaginitis. Symptoms include discharge, burning, itching, or vaginal soreness during intercourse.

Vaginal lubricants such as vegetable oil or unscented cold cream may help during intercourse. If not, the standard treatment is vaginal- or oral-conjugated estrogen (Premarin) daily for two or three weeks, then a maintenance schedule to prevent symptom recurrence. If a woman chooses vaginal estrogen cream instead of oral estrogen, she can use *very small amounts* (one-eighth of an applicator) two or three times per week. If the cream is used in small doses, there is little risk of systemic absorption. Women who do not want to use estrogen or women who have contraindications (e.g. history of breast cancer) may use a 1 percent testosterone cream vaginally. Apply a small amount to the sorest area at the vaginal entrance three times a week to reduce soreness and irritation.

Helping Yourself

Recurrent vaginitis is frustrating and can be costly. Experts agree that effective treatment relies on accurate diagnosis and treatment. Unfortunately, some clinicians make a di-

agnosis based only on the woman's discharge. Others diagnose on the results of a Pap smear. Addison says she sees numerous cases of "chronic vaginitis" that have simply recurred because they were misdiagnosed and mistreated to begin with.

"Some doctors," she says, "prescribe medication before it's clear what they are treating. You have to ascertain what's going on and what's causing the symptoms." Dr. Stewart agrees. She says the first task is to determine if it really is a chronic infection or if some other problem is causing the symptoms.

Sometimes treatment fails because the clinician uses a shotgun approach instead of the most effective medication. Other times, the infection is sexually transmitted and partners are not adequately treated.

For the most effective professional care:

- Do not douche or have intercourse for 48 hours before the exam. It hinders accurate diagnosis.
- Schedule a visit at a time other than your menstrual period. Menstrual flow makes diagnosis more difficult.
- Do not use "feminine hygiene" deodorant sprays on the vulva. They can cover up important indicators and increase discomfort.
- Request a "wet mount" or "wet smear." This involves mixing a sample of discharge with saline solution and examining it under a microscope. If the infectious agent is trichomonas or yeast, the clinician should be able to identify it. (Wet mounts are not conclusive for gonorrhea or chlamydia.)
- Request a gonorrhea culture. A culture is a good idea if a woman has a male partner who may have been with other partners, even if she has no symptoms. Women with gonorrhea typically show no symptoms, but if left untreated, the infection can cause potentially life-threatening pelvic inflammatory disease (PID).
- Request a chlamydia test, especially if you are a heterosexual woman with multiple sex partners. Chlamydia may be mistaken for vaginitis, but it can be diagnosed only with special tests.
- Have all sexual partners treated. Do not assume a part-

ner is infection-free because he or she doesn't have symptoms.

- Mention any drug allergies.
- Take all the prescribed medication. Symptoms often subside before the infection is completely cleared.
- Ask if you need a follow-up visit.
- If you are not satisfied with your treatment, seek a second opinion.

Some people believe that recurrent vaginitis is linked to our feelings about ourselves and our sexuality. Louise Hay, a therapist who works with chronically ill people and who is the author of *Heal Your Body and You Can Heal Your Life,* believes that illnesses, including vaginitis, are influenced by negative thoughts and feelings. "I see an enormous connection," says Hay, "between the mind's health and the body's. Women I've seen with chronic vaginitis often have frustrating relationships. They feel angry, but don't express their anger. Their genitals become the battleground for their unexpressed feelings." Hay recommends women with chronic vaginitis examine their relationships and their feelings about themselves.

Dr. Stewart says anything that causes stress compromises the body's ability to fight off infection and can help promote chronic vaginitis. "I've seen women who are going to law school or who are in the midst of a divorce," she says, "who suffer yeast infections over and over. When they graduate or the divorce becomes final and their stress level drops, their chronic infection clears up." Dr. Stewart says a high-sugar diet can also stress the body. "I've had women tell me their vaginitis cleared up when they stopped drinking 16 ounces of orange juice every morning."

Since lifestyle and personal habits may contribute to recurrent vaginitis, the following tips may help:

- Use unscented soap to keep the vaginal area clean because deodorant or perfumed soaps may irritate the vagina. Pat the vulva dry. Do not use others' towels or washcloths, because most vaginal infections can be spread by contact.
- Wear cotton underwear. This allows the vagina to

"breathe" and prevents the buildup of moisture and heat that support the growth of infectious organisms. Avoid nylon underwear and panty hose, unless they have a cotton panel in the crotch. Avoid very tight pants and change out of leotards and bathing suits promptly.

- Avoid bath oils, powders, bubble baths, and feminine hygiene sprays, which can irritate the skin around the vulva.
- Wipe from front to back. This avoids transporting anal bacteria into the vagina.
- Use K-Y Jelly or a bland vegetable oil, or contraceptive foam, cream, or jelly if you need extra lubrication during intercourse.
- Avoid routine douching. Douching may irritate and interfere with the vagina's normal ecosystem. If you are prone to recurrent infections, however, you might try acidifying the vagina with an occasional vinegar douche (1 to 3 tablespoons of vinegar to 1 quart of warm water).
- Take acidophilus tablets while taking antibiotics and afterward.
- If you are bothered by chronic vaginitis, use contraception other than the Pill, IUD, or contraceptive sponges. If you use a diaphragm, don't leave it in for more than 24 hours at a time.
- Use menstrual pads rather than tampons. Tampons, particularly superabsorbent brands, can interfere with the vagina's normal drainage. If you use tampons, change them at least three times a day, and alternate them with pads to allow the vagina to drain properly.
- Manage your stress load. Too much stress can alter the vagina's pH and lower the body's resistance to infection. If your vaginitis coincides with stressful events, consider slowing down, meditation, counseling, or other stress-management techniques. Regular exercise reduces stress and strengthens the body's overall resistance to illness.
- Avoid high-sugar foods. Too much sugar, dairy products, and artificial sweeteners alter the vaginal pH and provide food for infectious organisms. Eat a balanced low-fat, high-fiber diet that emphasizes whole grains, fresh fruits, and vegetables.

CHAPTER 27
Make Your Dermatitis Disappear

The perfume you safely use in the summer can "soak" into winter-dried skin and cause a rash.

What causes the red, itchy, scaly skin of allergic contact dermatitis? The answer may be at your fingertips. Or in your closet. Or in any one of a multitude of products you use regularly.

Allergens (the substances that trigger an allergic reaction) are found in common items we all touch daily. While most of us can splash on perfume, for example, without giving it a second thought, people who are sensitive to specific allergens may develop an unsightly and uncomfortable skin reaction. "A classic allergic reaction consists of dense blisters on red, swollen skin, as in poison ivy," says Albert M. Kligman, M.D., Ph.D., professor of dermatology at the University of Pennsylvania School of Medicine. "But in certain areas of your body, or in sensitive people who haven't been overly exposed to the allergen, these signs may be absent. That can make the allergy difficult to diagnose."

"One of the allergic contact dermatitis problems I see most often is flakiness and itching around the sensitive eye area," says Joseph Fowler, Jr., M.D., assistant professor of dermatology at the University of Louisville in Kentucky. "This reaction is usually caused by the fragrance or preservatives in cosmetics and lotions."

Dermatologists have to be part detective. If your eyes are puffy and itchy, eye makeup isn't the only suspect. The real culprit may be your nail polish. Most polishes contain fragrance and/or polymers, both common allergens. If

you're sensitive to those chemicals, all you have to do is brush your fingertips across your eyes or face, and the skin reacts.

There's another catch. "Many women come to me with a dermatitis condition around their eyes, and the first thing they tell me is that they couldn't be allergic to their eye cosmetics," says Dr. Fowler. "They've used the same brand for years with no trouble. But allergies just don't work that way. You can become sensitive to a substance at any time in your life."

If you have an allergy problem but don't feel dressed without your eye makeup or nail polish, a patch test can be done by your dermatologist to determine exactly which ingredient you're allergic to. Then it's up to you to read manufacturers' labels and avoid that ingredient.

One particularly troublesome allergen is formaldehyde. "Generalized dermatitis—itchy, flaky, red patches anywhere on the body—is often a reaction to formaldehyde," says Dr. Fowler. "It's a major undertaking to avoid formaldehyde, because it's in so very many things," he explains. "You may stop using cosmetics that contain formaldehyde and yet continue to have a skin problem. Few people realize that the chemical is released by such diverse agents as cigarette smoke and permanent-press fabrics. I've had patients with a terrible skin problem who quit smoking and got 90 percent better. Others changed their wardrobe to eliminate permanent-press clothing and had similar results."

Other reactions are equally subtle. Perhaps you're rubbing a medication or lotion on your skin to treat a minor burn. Yet the problem doesn't seem to go away in the time it should. See your doctor. Since injured skin is more easily sensitized, you could be experiencing a reaction to ingredients in the cream. Some common culprits: antibiotics (such as neomycin) and antimicrobial preservatives.

The Hot-Air Connection

If you suffer from allergic contact dermatitis, understanding how your skin functions can help you to help yourself.

Dry skin is more sensitive to irritants and allergens than

normal skin. As your skin loses moisture, it loses its ability to act as a barrier to allergens. "When your skin's moisture content drops, it becomes like a dry lake bed," says Edward K. Boisits, Ph.D., manager of biophysical research for the Erno Laszlo Institute in New York. "It soaks up any moisture it comes in contact with—including potential allergens like lanolin or perfume."

That's why the perfume you used last summer may not cause skin problems until you use it in the winter when your skin is dry. Then the ingredient to which you're allergic gets through your skin's barrier, and you have an allergic reaction. When we speak of the skin's barrier being broken, we don't necessarily mean that the break is visible as a scratch or redness. More often it simply appears dry. So keeping your skin's moisture level normal is a vital step toward healthy skin.

Two of your best allies in combating dry skin are a humidifier and a good moisturizer. "Room humidifiers are very effective," says Dr. Boisits, "but it's important to keep the unit clean and follow the manufacturer's instructions. And using a moisturizer should be an integral part of your skin-care routine."

Keep your skin-care routine as simple and gentle as possible. "Use the mildest soaps you can find," says Dr. Boisits. Use them on your body as well as your face. When you wash, don't scrub as though you were trying to wash off a layer of skin. Be gentle. And if you have dry skin, don't think you have to take a complete bath or shower every day, especially in cold weather.

After you bathe or wash, and your skin is well hydrated, pat dry and apply your moisturizer while your skin is slightly damp. "To help prevent chapped skin and dermatitis, use lotions regularly. Remember, the drier skin becomes, the more susceptible it is to allergens and irritants," says Dr. Boisits.

PART VII: MEN'S HEALTH NEWSFRONT

CHAPTER 28

Heart Disease and Exercise: No Pain, You Gain

You've read that eating *fish may benefit your heart; now research is showing that* going *fishing (and other leisure activities) may also prevent a heart attack.*

Steve is not a lazy man. He put a new roof on the garage last fall, and he plans to remodel the family room this summer. He also coaches Little League and keeps one of the tidiest yards in town.

What Steve does not do, however, is "exercise." At 5′10″ and 205 pounds, he would rather walk on hot coals than jog, he's too impatient to walk, and riding an exercise bike impresses him as a fate worse than atherosclerosis itself.

Is Steve a sitting duck for heart disease?

The question is a $64,000 one because as many as 90 percent of American men share Steve's situation—they're active but still do not get the minimum recommended dose of three 30-minute bouts of aerobic exercise a week. It's a demographic that forces you to wonder: Is there really such therapeutic magic to the aerobic prescription? Does

the heart really need to be revved regularly to stay in tune? Do the arteries need to be "flushed" regularly by accelerated blood flow to keep them supple and clear of life-threatening plaque?

Does working out, in short, have things to offer the heart that "work" does not? And what about nonphysical ways of reducing risks of heart disease? Can a nonexerciser make up for an exercise shortage by eating wisely, reducing stress, and keeping a tight lid on vice?

Strenuous Exercise Overrated

Ronald LaPorte, Ph.D., associate professor in the Department of Epidemiology at the University of Pittsburgh,

Burning Calories around the House

The following activities, done on a daily basis, can be substituted for more strenuous forms of aerobic exercise in the prevention of heart disease, new research suggests. A daily minimum of 30 to 70 minutes is recommended. The "calories burned" figures are for someone who weighs 180 to 200 pounds.

Activity	Calories Burned per Hour
Work	
Bricklaying	235
Carpentry	
light	200–270
heavy	415
Chopping wood	
by hand	525
with a power saw	260
Cleaning windows	295
Gardening (hoeing, digging)	400–450
Hanging clothes on a clothesline	285–300
House painting	245

fielded that bevy of questions this way: "Research is now suggesting that the value of strenuous exercise in the prevention of heart disease may be overrated. Yes, exercise can favorably modify all the major risk factors for heart disease—blood pressure, serum cholesterol, high glucose levels, body fat, and possibly even potentially harmful levels of hormones brought on by stress. But the amount and intensity of exercise needed to do this appears to be considerably less than had been thought.

"We know now, too, that all the major risk factors for heart disease can be modified in other ways—serum cholesterol through diet, for example, and blood pressure through diet and relaxation techniques. I'm afraid the fitness movement has done the average man a disservice with its credo of 'no pain, no gain.' It's very possible,

Activity	**Calories Burned per Hour**
Pushing a power mower	310
Scrubbing floors	295
Shoveling snow	710
Stacking wood	400–440
Washing and polishing a car	270
Play	
Bowling	240
Dancing	300–450
Fishing (wading)	350
Golf	
twosome, carrying clubs	440
twosome, puling clubs	385
foursome, carrying clubs	310
foursome, pulling clubs	295
Horseback riding	
walk	195
trot	475
Piano playing	145
Ping-Pong	525
Sex	155–350
Tennis	
singles	495
doubles	350

indeed, to have a healthy heart without being aerobically fit in the clinical sense of the word."

The research to which Dr. LaPorte refers includes the latest chapter of the ongoing MRFIT (multiple risk factor intervention trial) currently being done with 12,000 middle-aged men in Minneapolis. Latest results show that men who regularly engage in light to moderate physical activity (e.g., gardening, yard work, home repairs, walking, bowling, and even *fishing*) enjoy essentially the same protection from heart disease as men whose activity levels are considerably higher. Men who expended a modest average of 224 calories a day in leisure-time activities were found to be as well protected from fatal heart attacks as men who expended an average of nearly three times that much.

Consistency Is Key

The key to benefiting from these activities, however, appeared to be engaging in them on a regular basis for 30 to 70 minutes daily.

"The message we're getting is that regularity may be more important than intensity," Dr. LaPorte says. "If you can putter around the house or yard for between 30 and 70 minutes a day, you may be doing your heart as much good as you would by going to the gym three times a week."

Hear that, Steve? Go ahead and remodel the family room this summer, but don't be afraid to break up the job. Better to do 45 to 60 minutes daily for a month and then move on to something else rather than blitzing the job in a week and then lying idle. "Work around the house can be a great form of exercise," Dr. LaPorte says. "But too often, men make it erratic or seasonal. If activities around the house and yard are going to be your form of exercise, be as consistent as possible. Try to do something for at least 45 minutes every day rather than working all day just on weekends or on your vacation. The body prefers consistency to surprise."

CHAPTER 29
A Man's Guide to Weight Loss

Differences between the sexes call for different plans of action to lose weight.

Thirty years ago you could take a Ralph Kramden physique to a backyard swimming party and actually show the thing off. Size stood for durability and power, in cars and men alike, so why *not* a few cannonballs to broadcast your worth?

But then came the fitness movement, and advances in the understanding of heart disease, and Jim Palmer posing in his jockey shorts. Needless to say, the Ralph Kramden look now feels more comfortable back by the barbeque in a kimono.

Brando's No Match for Rambo

"It's a whole new set of standards and pressures men now find themselves faced with," says Michael R. Lowe, Ph.D., director of the Weight Management Program at Temple University. "Men today feel a much greater obligation to be trim and athletic, not just because of urgings from the medical community but because of the new, more muscular images of masculinity being presented by movies, TV, and the fashion industry."

The effect of this muscular onslaught from the media? "Men are beginning to share many of the same fat preoccupations as women," claims Adam Drewnowski, Ph.D., University of Michigan assistant professor of nutrition and psychology.

As many as 10 percent of the nation's bulimics (frequent binge-eaters who vomit or purge themselves with laxatives) may now be men. And when Dr. Drewnowski sur-

veyed a recent incoming class of freshmen at the University of Michigan, he found that virtually all the men were unhappy with their physique in some way.

"About half wanted to be thinner, while the other half wanted more muscular bulk," Dr. Drewnowski says.

But is this new obsession with physique a hang-up of the younger breed only? No fan of Teddy Roosevelt would ever get pushed out of shape about a little extra "latitude." Right?

Wrong. Dr. Drewnowski suspects some older men may be even *more* fat conscious because of the health hazards now linked with middle-age obesity. "It's my guess that many older men may feel a double pressure—the cosmetic as well as the medical," he says.

Lean Is Masculine

Health and fashion aside, there may be yet another reason that today's Ralph Kramden is less comfortable about throwing his weight around: The equalization of the sexes is putting greater pressure on men to show their muscle as a way of showing their masculinity.

"Changing sex roles have made the body the last bastion of difference between men and women and thus even more closely tied to self-image and sense of identity," says Yale University professor of psychology and psychiatry Judith Rodin, Ph.D.

Muscle, in short, is making something of a caveman comeback as a distinguishing factor between the sexes. An athletic physique for a man now approaches the prestigious job, big house, and exotic car as a sign of accomplishment and male worth, Dr. Rodin says.

A far cry, certainly, from the days when a big splash at the pool was the only resumé a real man needed.

Exploit Your Male Advantage

So the days of respectable rotundity have gone the way of the brontosaurus. What's a guy with girth to do?

"Men are notorious, unfortunately, for doing too little or too much," says Art Mollen, D.O., founder and medical

director of the Southwest Health Institute. "If they're not spending weekends watching sporting events on TV and drinking beer, they're fasting or sweating bullets in a rubber sweat suit."

"Men are great at losing weight when they decide they want to," agrees Dr. Lowe. "The problem is getting men motivated to start on a weight-loss program in the first place."

So how's this for incentive: Weight control is not only more important for men, it's *easier*. Research leaves little doubt that fat weighs more heavily on the male heart, but the good news is that the male body is not only more resistant to gaining weight, it's also better at *losing* it!

"Men have a higher percentage of muscle than women, so they burn more calories even at rest," Dr. Mollen says. "The male sex hormone testosterone, moreover, encourages the development of muscles. The female sex hormone estrogen encourages the development of fat. Men enjoy weight-control advantages over women that are as basic as the genes."

That being the case, it's high time an estimated one-fifth of American men brought their genes out of retirement. That's how many men are more than 20 percent overweight and hence endangering their health as well as their egos.

Set Your Sights on Your Setpoint

Even for this crowd, however, weight-loss experts are now issuing words of warning. "Don't strive for a weight that's going to be a lifelong struggle to maintain. You're only programming yourself for failure if you do."

Those words come from Richard Keesey, Ph.D., a professor of psychology at the University of Wisconsin in Madison and originator of the "setpoint" theory of weight regulation. "The body has a certain weight that it prefers for a number of complex biological reasons," Dr. Keesey says. "To attempt to go below that weight is to ask for inadvisable physical as well as psychological consequences."

As you begin to lose weight, fewer calories are burned

because the body weighs less and thus requires less energy for any given motion. And metabolism slows down, leading to a further recession in calorie burning. The result is that food becomes, in a sense, more "fattening."

Put those two phenomena together and you've got the foundation of the setpoint theory. "It's the body's way of keeping weight from falling below a healthy level," says Dr. Keesey.

Research shows that eating disorders, fatigue, depression, and impaired circulation can result from trying to achieve a weight that, biologically speaking, is just not in the cards.

"Diet is a form of starvation," adds Harvard Medical School professor of psychiatry James I. Hudson, M.D. "Your body is fighting back." An eating binge, for example, can be triggered by attempting to diet to as little as 10 percent below your set body weight, Dr. Hudson says.

But setpoint physiology works in the other direction, too, by discouraging *obesity* just as it discourages emaciation, Dr. Keesey says.

Proof of that pudding is the perspiration on your forehead after a third helping of Aunt Gertrude's mince pie. "Overeating steps up metabolism, which steps up calorie burning, which produces body heat," Dr. Keesey explains. "It's all part of the setpoint mechanism—the body's biological effort to weigh what it should *despite* dietary indiscretions from us."

All of which raises the $64,000 question, of course, of just what that "most natural weight" is.

Let Your Blood Be Your Guide

"This may disappoint those who hope that down deep they're supposed to be built like Richard Gere, but probably the best way to determine whether you're at your best weight is simply to get a physical—one that includes a blood test," Dr. Keesey says. "If your blood pressure, cholesterol, triglycerides, and blood sugar levels are all normal, you're probably as close to your ideal weight as you need to be."

Despite what the weight charts say?

Yes, despite what the weight charts say. "There's too much variation in the way people are constructed, men especially, for those charts to be taken as the final word," Dr. Keesey says.

Boxer Mike Tyson, for example, probably would be obese according to standardized weight charts, when in truth little of that weight is fat, Dr. Keesey says.

And what if your blood test reveals results that are *not* normal?

You should get your doctor's opinion, of course, but Dr. Keesey's advice is to try three basic changes in lifestyle: less fat, more fiber, and more regular exercise.

Exactly how long such a regimen takes to bring you and your setpoint together depends on the weight you're starting from, Dr. Keesey says, but his advice is to not be overly anxious.

If pounds have been years in the making, they're not going to be overnight in the taking, Dr. Keesey and other experts agree. The longer weight loss takes, in fact, the longer it's apt to last.

Exercise Makes Perfect Sense

Where does exercise fit into the body's quest for its ideal weight?

It can be just the push your metabolism needs. Dieting's shortcoming in weight loss is that it slows the metabolism, but exercise has just the opposite effect: It boosts calorie burning as you *do* it, and studies suggest it may keep the ovens burning for several hours afterward. Add a *muscle-building* component to your exercise program, and you really put fat on the skillet.

"Aerobic exercise (e.g., walking, jogging, cycling, and swimming) is great for burning calories and conditioning the heart," says Dr. Mollen. "But by adding a muscle-building segment to your program, you get a calorie-burning partner that's with you all the time."

But exercise goes beyond even calorie burning in the battle of the bulge, says Jerome D. Cohen, M.D., of the St. Louis University School of Medicine.

"Exercise lowers insulin levels, and since one of the roles

of insulin is to facilitate fat storage, the person who exercises regularly is impeding this process."

Better yet, Dr. Cohen emphasizes that activity far short of the sweat-making kind is capable of producing such metabolic benefits. "Walking, lawn work, gardening, taking stairs instead of an escalator—any activity that raises heart rate above a sedentary level—is going to burn fat and help tune the metabolism."

And it's going to benefit the spirit as well. "I'm convinced that the psychological rewards of an active lifestyle are as important in weight control as the physical effects," Dr. Cohen says. "When a man's active, he feels better about himself, so he's going to be less attracted to self-defeating behaviors such as overindulgence in food and drink."

The rules of the fat-fighting program are threefold: Think about exercise *frequency* more than intensity, supplement aerobic activity with muscle building, and consider *any* activity better than no activity at all.

Frequency. "You want to get your body into a higher calorie-burning gear, and the more frequently you exercise, the better your chances of doing that," Dr. Mollen says. "Try to do something aerobic for at least 10 minutes *every day.* Thirty minutes would be better, of course, but consistency should be your primary goal. If you can eat every day, you can exercise every day."

Muscle building. "Nothing fancy here either," Dr. Mollen says. "You can join the local health club for their weight machines if you want, but push-ups, sit-ups, and chin-ups can build muscle just about as well."

And by building muscle, remember, you're boosting the rate at which your body burns calories—even at rest. "Do some sort of strength training three days a week," Dr. Mollen says.

Activity in general. "Too many men think they have to be in a sweat suit to be burning calories," says Dr. Cohen. "They fail to realize the value of such things as taking the stairs instead of the elevator or cutting the grass with a push mower instead of a ride-on. It's the *grand total* of calories we burn that dictates weight control, not just those isolated few we manage to squeeze into formal workouts."

Have Your "Cake" and Weight Loss, Too

"Give men the option of eating less or exercising more to lose weight, and they'll usually choose the exercise route," says Dr. Lowe. "Women, on the other hand, usually opt for dieting."

Which road is the wiser one to travel?

If you could choose only one, probably exercise, Dr. Lowe says. "Dieting without exercise risks loss of muscle tissue, and a would-be weight loser certainly doesn't want that."

Research indicates, too, that weight loss via exercise results in more favorable changes in blood fats: HDL (those heart-helping high-density lipoproteins) gets a boost, while LDL (villainous low-density lipoproteins) gets a boot. Dieting alone usually results in decreases in HDL and LDL alike.

But before you cycle off to the pizzeria with that news, keep in mind that eating better—and notice we didn't say eating *less*—can facilitate a weight-loss program immensely.

"The key to making weight loss as healthful and as easy as possible is to get diet and exercise working in tandem," Dr. Lowe said. "Fat will be lost faster, muscle tissue will be spared, and health will be optimally enhanced."

So here we go: dieting tips best suited for getting that fat-burning tandem in gear.

Don't go on a diet—fix the one you've got. The biggest mistake most men make in dieting is that they bite off more than they can chew, says Bryant Stamford, Ph.D., director of the Health Promotion and Wellness Center at the University of Louisville School of Medicine.

"When you make a dietary change, ask yourself whether you'll be able to keep with it for the next ten years," he says. If not, it may be too extreme. Better to ease into a more healthful style of eating gradually than to try to become a convert overnight, Dr. Stamford says.

Remember that the longer weight loss takes, the longer it's apt to last. "You shouldn't try to lose weight faster than about 1 percent of your existing body weight

per week," says Theodore Van Itallie, M.D., of St. Luke's/ Roosevelt Hospital in New York. For a 200-pounder, that's no more than 2 pounds a week. Go faster than that and you risk more than making yourself miserable—your body could flip into what weight-loss experts call the "starvation response," where the body conserves fat as it would during a famine.

Consider dietary fat your worst enemy. Fat not only beats protein and carbohydrates in the calorie department (by more than two to one; fat contains 9 calories per gram compared with about 4 for carbos and protein) but also is a proven no-no for the heart. And it's downright eager to turn into flab: Only one-fifth as much energy is required of the digestive system to convert dietary fat into body fat as is required for carbohydrates, for example. Add the fact that saturated fat (the kind in butter, cheese, whole milk, and meat) seems especially inclined to deposit its excess calories in the area of the abdomen, and you'll want to think twice before buttering that next piece of bread, for sure.

Consider dietary fiber your best friend. High-fiber foods are more filling: Research suggests that fiber may actually help *erase* calories from other foods by sweeping them through the intestines before they've had a chance to be digested. Studies show, too, that certain types of fiber are effective at lowering blood fats and blood pressure and reducing the risk of colon cancer.

Throw away your scale. Or at least hide it, Dr. Stamford says. Frequent weigh-ins can confuse a weight-loss campaign by showing temporary fluctuations such as water retention or *positive* situations such as muscle gain. "You have to change your thinking from weight loss to *fat* loss," Dr. Stamford says. Simply looking in a mirror or keeping track of your waist size can tell you more about your progress than any scale.

Count satisfaction, not just calories. If a lunch of coffee and crackers is going to have you bulldozing your way through your refrigerator the minute you get home, what good is it? But keeping satisfied is important not just for avoiding binges but also for keeping weight loss working metabolically. The body reacts to extreme hunger by

putting the brakes on calorie burning—so pull calories from your diet in ways your body is least likely to notice, suggests Brigham Young University exercise physiologist Garth Fischer, Ph.D. Try a leaner cut of steak or a light beer instead of the real thing. And speaking of the sauce . . .

Be realistic about alcohol. Alcohol's calories may not have the fat-producing equivalent of the calories in food (that was the verdict reached by a recent study in the *Journal of the American College of Nutrition*), but alcohol has other effects that can make it fattening indeed, as anyone who's ever gone through an entire pepperoni pizza during a night of merrymaking can sadly attest. Keeping a lid on your drinking may help you keep a lid on your eating.

Expect plateaus. They're a natural part of the weight-loss process and should not be cause for disillusionment or concern, says Dr. Van Itallie. Weight loss will resume as soon as the body has had a chance to make certain necessary metabolic adjustments.

Do not seesaw. It's okay and perhaps even advisable to take occasional vacations from a weight-loss effort—periods where you maintain rather than continue to lose—but do not backslide. Research now shows that weight loss may get more difficult each time you do it, so do yourself the favor of doing it just once.

CHAPTER 30

Nine New Treatments for Male Infertility

From bed to surgical table, doctors tell what can be done for virtually every man with this problem.

"Just relax!" "Eat asparagus!" "Try acupuncture!"

A man who is trying in vain to father a child is apt to hear all sorts of cockamamie advice. Most of it, however well-intentioned, is useless. Still, there *is* such a thing as good advice. In fact, says Neil Baum, M.D., director of the New Orleans Male Infertility Clinic, "as a result of advances over the past two decades, physicians are entering an exciting era in which we have something of therapeutic value to offer virtually every patient who has an infertility problem."

"Home Remedies"

What are these discoveries? Well, the remedies range from high tech to homespun, from the ridiculously simple to the sublime.

Try Taking Robitussin

The active ingredient in many over-the-counter expectorants (quanifenesin) seems to make semen thinner and less viscous, enabling sperm to more easily reach and fertilize an egg, says Marc Cohen, M.D., clinical associate professor of urology at New York University Medical Center. Dr. Cohen's work correlates with the discovery in 1981 by Jerome H. Check, M.D., a fertility specialist at Thomas Jefferson University Hospital in Philadelphia, that Robitussin thins cervical mucus, making it easier for sperm to penetrate and reach an egg.

"This discovery is so recent that I haven't had a chance to organize a controlled scientific study," says Dr. Cohen. "But I tell my patients to try it, and I know it helps the sperm, although it's too soon to say how many pregnancies have resulted.

"I also have these men take 500 milligrams of vitamin C three times a day, to acidify the semen and facilitate the process," he says.

Watch Your Timing

Your chances of initiating pregnancy can be increased by timing intercourse to coincide with ovulation. (It's sort of like turning the rhythm method of birth control on its head.) A new urine test can predict ovulation more accurately than the basal body temperature test that many infertile couples currently use.

"Sperm remains in the female genital tract for 48 hours after intercourse," explains Dr. Baum. "But if you have intercourse too frequently—once a day or more—the sperm count will be lower. So, ideally, a couple that is trying to conceive should have intercourse on the day of ovulation, as well as two days before and afterward."

"I had one patient, a dentist, who was in the middle of working on his mother's teeth when his wife telephoned that the time was right," recalls one doctor. "He dropped everything and left his mother waiting in the chair while he raced home, made love to his wife, and drove back to the office; he then finished the dental work on his mother." (Love on demand paid off: His wife got pregnant.)

Make Love Twice in One Hour

A study published in the journal *Fertility and Sterility* reports that 14 out of 20 men with low sperm counts who tried this had higher sperm counts in the second ejaculation. Five of their wives became pregnant. Anthony Thomas, M.D., who heads the male infertility section of the Department of Urology at the Cleveland Clinic Foundation, notes that with this method, stronger, fresher sperm may be ejaculated the second time around.

Sexual Science

If all the simple things fail, you may have to consult a fertility specialist—usually a urologist, endocrinologist, or other physician with experience in treating infertility. Here are some of the promising new weapons in their arsenal.

Varicocele Surgery

Varicose veins in the scrotum—*varicoceles* (VAR-i-ko-seels)—are thought to be the most common cause of male infertility. Found in 30 to 40 percent of infertile men, these enlarged veins are believed to interfere with fertility by supplying too much blood to the scrotum, thereby overheating the testes. A varicocele feels like a "bag of worms" beneath the soft skin of the scrotum.

Standard treatment for varicoceles, used for about the last 40 years, is surgery. The doctor makes an incision in the scrotum under general anesthesia or, more recently, local anesthesia, ties off the veins, and then stitches you back up. You're in the hospital for one day, can resume nonphysical activity in three to five days, and physical work or play in two to three weeks. You'll have a Demerol injection and will probably need painkillers for 48 hours. Cost varies from region to region, but runs about $1,500. Results vary, too: Sperm quality improves in 53 to 92 percent of patients, with a subsequent pregnancy rate of 30 to 55 percent, according to a report in *Postgraduate Medicine*.

Balloon Insertion

In a newer, nonsurgical procedure called percutaneous venographic occlusion, the offending vein is simply plugged up with a tiny balloon or coil. A radiologist slips a catheter into a leg vein through a puncture in the skin, then guides the catheter into position. When it's seated inside the proper vein, the doctor implants the balloon through the catheter.

"The advantage of this method over standard varicocele repair is that it requires no incision, so postoperative recuperation is shorter," says Dr. Baum. "There is no discomfort or pain, so no medication is needed, and you can

return to full activity in two or three days. The costs are about the same.

"The *disadvantage* is that the balloon or coil can migrate to the lungs and cause an embolism [life-threatening blockage of a blood vessel]. So many doctors and their patients opt for standard surgery, turning to balloon or coil insertion if surgery fails and the varicoceles are still present."

Microsurgery

With the aid of optical microscopes, doctors can surgically open up sperm ductwork obstructed by infections or congenital defects. "Microsurgery in the male reproductive tract is relatively new—much newer than in the female," says Larry Lipshultz, M.D., professor of urology at Baylor College of Medicine in Houston.

After microsurgery for vasectomy reversal, sperm show up in semen 90 percent of the time but are present less frequently after surgery for other reasons. Reported pregnancy rates vary from 45 to 70 percent. Pregnancy occurs within as few as nine or ten months in many cases, Dr. Lipshultz says. The surgeon's fee alone may run from $2,000 to $6,000, making this one of the more expensive treatments for male infertility.

Ofloxacin

This is a new antibacterial drug found to be effective against sexually transmitted organisms, including chlamydia and gonorrhea. Infections are an increasingly common cause of infertility in men who stayed in sexual circulation for an extended spell before settling down to marriage or monogamy. Ofloxacin works against organisms that have become resistant to penicillin, tetracycline, or spectinomycin.

Sperm Washing

This can be used to improve the velocity of sluggish sperm by washing away seminal plasma. Sperm are placed in a special protein-enriched medium for 15 or 20 minutes. The strongest sperm are separated from the weakest, then introduced into the womb via artificial insemination.

Electrically Stimulated Ejaculation

"This is a brand-new technique—developed within the past year," says Dr. Lipshultz. "It's exciting because it makes fatherhood possible for men who until now could not ejaculate or have an erection due to spinal cord injury or lymph-adenectomy [removal of lymph nodes]." So far, six pregnancies have resulted.

All this takes patience.

"Some men want to know the odds for pregnancy the minute their sperm leave their penis," says Dr. Baum. But most efforts to improve sperm take a minimum of three months, because it takes 90 days for a new sperm to be produced, reach maturity, and report for duty. All told, the evaluation and treatment of male infertility may take a year or two—or longer—and run into thousands of dollars. And while the chances of success for each method are rarely 100 percent, says Dr. Thomas, if you add them all up, the odds can look pretty good.

Then all you have to do is figure out how to diaper a baby.

CHAPTER 31

A Guide to Cosmetic Surgery for Men

Doctors discuss the right and wrong reasons for wanting a surgically improved appearance.

Would Clark Gable have allowed anyone to monkey with his ears? Would Winston Churchill have surrendered to a chin tuck? Would John Wayne have let his crow's-feet be scalped?

It seems sheer heresy to think so.

But that was then and now is now. The "me-ism" of the past 20 years has lured male vanity out of the closet as never before. Roughly 30 percent of all cosmetic surgeries now are being performed on men, and the numbers are growing. Could it be time for *you* to sacrifice pride for a more sightly hide?

Maybe and maybe not, the experts say. As important as what you want done is *why* you want it done. If a new personality is what you're after, forget it. "Cosmetic surgery doesn't change personality—it changes appearance. A person must want physical rather than psychological results," says Mary Ruth Wright, Ph.D., a professor at the Baylor College of Medicine in Houston. "A man can be very dissatisfied if his decision to have cosmetic surgery is based on factors other than his appearance."

John Goin, M.D., agrees. "The patient is lying on an operating table, not a couch," says Dr. Goin, clinical professor of surgery at the University of Southern California School of Medicine and coauthor of *Changing the Body: Psychological Effects of Cosmetic Surgery.* "If a person's motivations are wrong—if he has irrational or magical expectations—that person will be made psychologically worse by the operation."

Be Realistic

Which isn't to say that cosmetic alteration doesn't have things to offer, however. Dr. Goin says the best reason for cosmetic surgery is simply to bring your looks more in line with your attitudes and goals.

"When someone notices the development of age-related changes and says, 'I'm not really that person in the mirror. I feel younger than that, and I want to look how I feel,' that's a realistic motive for cosmetic surgery."

Wanting a little help up the career ladder qualifies as a motive, too, Dr. Goin says. "I don't think it's true that cosmetic surgery will improve everybody's career—the world is filled with haggard-looking business executives who are doing wonderfully well—but it can work for a

Making the Right Decision

If you're thinking about having cosmetic surgery, doctors emphasize that you must do some self-examination to determine your motivation. Here are some examples of reasons that they feel are valid, and some that should prompt you to reconsider.

Right Reasons

- To correct an obvious physical deformity.
- To improve an already basically positive self-image.
- To increase chances of career advancement.
- To look less tired or more youthful.
- To boost self-confidence.

Wrong Reasons

- To improve a personal relationship.
- To elevate low self-esteem.
- To relieve grief.
- To satisfy someone else.
- To stop Father Time in his tracks.

man who feels he needs it." Cosmetic surgery often can give just a little extra boost of confidence.

But notice the word "extra." There's no way cosmetic surgery can turn a Walter Mitty into a Donald Trump. And it's not going to rehabilitate any sagging personal relationships either. "If a guy thinks, 'My girlfriend left me for a better-looking man. Maybe if I have a face lift, I'll get her back,' that kind of motivation will almost always end in disappointment," Dr. Goin says.

Also ill-fated is the "sudden hatred" syndrome, Dr. Goin says. "When a man has been walking around with a certain nose for 50 years and suddenly decides to change it, he has motivations that are less than realistic."

Be Specific

It's also important to be *specific* about what you want accomplished by surgery, Dr. Goin says, which is something that men more than women may find difficult. "Women tend to see their body parts distinctly—their ears, their eyes, their hands. Men, however, tend to see their bodies globally—all at once. So a man should focus on *exactly* which feature he wants to improve. He shouldn't say, 'I just want to look better.' Does he want the bags removed from his eyes? Does he want a nose job because his nose makes him look different from other people?" He should be as exact as possible in articulating his needs.

Also unlikely to succeed is any surgery motivated by desperation, Dr. Wright and Dr. Goin agree. Grief, depression, extremely low self-esteem, a failing marriage—these are problems for a psychiatrist, not a surgeon.

Who's Getting What

Below are descriptions of the most common operations performed on men in 1986 by members of the American Society of Plastic and Reconstructive Surgeons.

Nose Surgery (Rhinoplasty)

Whether your nose is bent, bumpy, or big, the operation is basically the same. You're sedated and given a local or general anesthetic (standard operating procedure for all cosmetic surgery). The surgeon goes in through the nostrils and makes incisions inside the nose, which is why there is no visible scar. He or she separates skin from bones and goes to work. If it's a bump, the surgeon saws it away and brings the nasal bones together to make a narrower bridge. If a new tip is what's wanted, he or she removes cartilage and reshapes the nose. For a smaller nose, the bones are chiseled into shape.

Number performed on men: 20,558.
Percentage performed on men: 25 percent.
Cost: $1,500 to $6,000.

Eyelid Surgery (Blepharoplasty)

This is really a fat-removal operation: The surgeon makes incisions under and over the eyes and removes the fat pads. This gets rid of bags under your eyes and folds of skin over them.

Number performed on men: 15,244.
Percentage performed on men: 18 percent.
Cost: $1,000 to $4,000.

Dermabrasion

This procedure is actually sophisticated sandpapering to remove scars. The skin (derma) is abraded off, and new, smoother skin grows back. It can't remove your old girlfriend's name from your bicep, though. Also, it's not a treatment for active acne—but it can help smooth and even out acne-scarred skin.

Number performed on men: 7,096.
Percentage performed on men: 27 percent.
Cost: $250 to $2,500.

Face Lift

The C-shaped incision around the front of each ear runs from your hairline to the back of your neck. The skin is pulled off the muscles and bones and lifted back. The excess skin is cut off. Another incision is made under your chin, and the fat there is removed.

Number performed on men: 6,693.
Percentage performed on men: 10 percent.
Cost: $2,000 to $10,000.

Ear Surgery (Otoplasty)

Most men have this operation because their ears don't have normal folds and so appear bowl-shaped and prominent. For this problem, the surgeon makes an incision behind the ears, weakens the cartilage, and puts in stitches so that the ear folds properly. Other operations correct protruding ears, ears that fold at the top, pointy ears—and any other strange shape you can imagine.

Number performed on men: 6,547.
Percentage performed on men: 44 percent.
Cost: $1,000 to $3,500.

Body-Fat Reduction (Lipectomy)

This is like maid service for your fat: The surgeon vacuums the areas you didn't have the time or energy to clean up yourself—thighs, abdomen, buttocks, you name it. The vacuum in this case is a cannula, a thin tube that's inserted through an incision and sucks the fat out.

Number performed on men: 5,966.
Percentage performed on men: 6 percent.
Cost: $500 to $4,000.

Hair Transplant

The surgeon removes plugs of hair follicles and transplants them in receded areas, or may operate on the entire scalp, slicing it open and pulling it over so that the areas on the sides where hair still grows are now on top. It's important to shop around and find a surgeon with a track record of producing natural-looking hairlines.

Number performed on men: 2,800
Percentage performed on men: 95 percent.
Cost: $250 to $4,000.

Chin Augmentation (Mentoplasty)

To improve a protruding or receding chin, the surgeon works from inside the mouth. He or she cuts through the bone and moves the chin, wiring it into its desired position. In the case of a receding chin, the surgeon may insert a plastic implant.

Number performed on men: 2,759.
Percentage performed on men: 18 percent.
Cost: $250 to $3,000.

Tummy Tuck (Abdominoplasty)

This procedure gets rid of flabby stomach muscles and loose abdominal skin. The surgeon makes an incision from hipbone to hipbone, lifts the skin, tightens the abdominal muscles and tissue with sutures, pulls the skin down, cuts off the excess, and closes the incision. Somewhere in there, he or she builds a new belly button, too.

Number performed on men: 2,264.
Percentage performed on men: 7 percent.
Cost: $2,000 to $6,000.

PART VIII: MEDICAL ADVANCES FOR A MORE BEAUTIFUL YOU

CHAPTER 32
Look Younger with Alpha Hydroxy Acids

This promising treatment for acne, age spots, and wrinkles is based on something as natural as a fruit.

Cosmetic companies usually get the pleasure of announcing new anti-aging skin-care treatments. But this time the medical community has the honor. The American Academy of Dermatology has unveiled a promising new anti-aging skin treatment: alpha hydroxy acids.

A family of natural compounds found in plants, fruits, and sour milk, alpha hydroxy acids may hold the key to smoother, younger-looking skin. In preliminary studies, they reduced wrinkles, faded age spots, improved dry skin, and helped reduce acne and acne scarring.

The leading researcher and authority on alpha hydroxy acids, Eugene J. Van Scott, M.D., clinical professor of dermatology at Temple University in Philadelphia, has used alpha hydroxy acids for 15 years to treat acne and ichthyosis (from the Greek word for fish; a disorder character-

ized by extremely dry and scaly skin). He noticed that during the course of these treatments, some of his patients began to look younger. Their age spots faded. In some cases, wrinkles seemed to disappear. Clearly, something was happening. But what?

Erasing Age Spots

In many skin conditions, including acne, dead skin cells don't slough off as they should. They accumulate on the skin's surface, forming a thick outer layer. "If you can eliminate the buildup of these dead cells, the skin improves," says Dr. Van Scott. "And that's how alpha hydroxy acids help. They soften the 'physiological glue' that holds the skin's dead surface cells together."

Further, Dr. Van Scott theorizes, alpha hydroxy acids may work on age spots the same way they work on acne. There are two types of age spots: One looks like a raised, scaly brown patch; the other looks like freckles. Both respond well to this treatment.

"For the raised brown patches, I apply a high concentration of alpha hydroxy acids. Within a minute or so, the thick raised layer of skin softens and begins to separate from the normal skin below. I can then gently lift it off," he explains. "When treating the freckle type of age spot, I use a combination of alpha hydroxy acid and a bleaching agent. This treatment is done more slowly, over a period of weeks. The spot gradually fades."

Wrinkle Removal

Dr. Van Scott also reports promising results with alpha hydroxy acids on fine lines and wrinkles. The treatment itself is a very simple office procedure. The alpha hydroxy acid concentration is applied to the skin for a few minutes, then rinsed off with water. "The patient may feel a little sting, which tells us a certain amount of the concentration is getting through the skin and having its effect," he says.

Admittedly, he does not yet know exactly how these compounds affect wrinkles. Also, more research is needed to determine what concentrations produce the best results,

how long the results will last, and whether the treatment will work equally well for everyone.

A six-month study of specific alpha hydroxy acids should resolve these unanswered questions. Testing is under way.

"Based on our observations so far, we feel that it's a fact that alpha hydroxy acids can reduce wrinkles," says Dr. Van Scott. "But we don't yet know the details."

For Professional Use Only

Keep in mind that, because alpha hydroxy acids cause a change in the structure of the skin, they are available only through a dermatologist or other physician. It's unlikely that home treatments using the natural plant source would be successful. "Fruits or plants don't contain the concentration of alpha hydroxy acid we use clinically," says Dr. Van Scott.

What can we expect for the future? If further studies confirm preliminary findings, alpha hydroxy acid treatment may supplant the face lift.

CHAPTER 33

Better Looks and Better Vision with Cosmetic Eye Surgery

A surgeon explains what's available and how it's done.

Ellen recently confided to a friend that she was going to have cosmetic surgery on her eyes. Why? Because she'd realized that she was wearing sunglasses everywhere, to hide eyes that look 20 years older than the rest of her. To be more accurate, her eyes are fine. It's the skin around them that's loose and baggy.

Ellen isn't alone with this problem. Factors such as heredity, prolonged sun exposure, and excessive swelling caused by allergies often combine to prematurely age and distort this most delicate area.

For some other people, however, it's not primarily a cosmetic problem that leads them to cosmetic surgery. Sagging folds of eyelid skin can actually weigh so heavily on the eyelid that partially blocked vision and eyestrain result.

Once you've decided to correct the problem, what's actually involved in cosmetic surgery around the eyes?

The doctor first determines which treatment to use. "The procedure depends on the type of problem the patient has," says Samuel J. Stegman, M.D., associate clinical professor of dermatology at the University of California at San Francisco. "People with wrinkles from sun damage, for instance, are often best treated with a chemical peel. But if the problem is heavy, saggy eyelids caused by excess skin or fat, eyelid surgery called blepharoplasty is needed to relieve the problem."

Lifting the Lids

"A blepharoplasty is usually done as an office procedure," says Dr. Stegman. "First I mark the area in pen, with the patient sitting and talking to me so that I can see what's involved. This way I can show the patient what I'll be doing during surgery and what he or she can expect.

"During the procedure itself, I prefer to use local anesthesia so that the patient is awake and able to move the eyes," continues Dr. Stegman. "I'll have the patient look to the ceiling and open his or her mouth to be sure how much skin is really excess and how much is needed for freedom of movement.

"This isn't absolutely necessary, though—the procedure can even be done under general anesthesia. Or if a patient is very tense, we can administer a mild sedative that will wear off quickly," he assures. "Some people are afraid to be awake because they're squeamish about the blood. Actually, there's very little bleeding.

"During a blepharoplasty on the lower lid, the incision is made just under the lash line, while on the upper lid, it is made in the fold," says Dr. Stegman. "The doctor then assesses how much skin, muscle, and fat need to be removed without compromising the eye's movement. The doctor excises it and sutures the skin. This all takes from 45 minutes to an hour for either the upper or lower eyelids.

"Afterward, I ask the patient to rest for 24 to 48 hours—which means no TV or reading. Then comes mild activity and wearing sunglasses for three to five days, until the stitches come out. There may be some bruising and swelling, which can last from less than a day to two weeks, although some people might take longer. Generally, if you are taking time off from work, a week is enough."

Don't Be Browbeaten

Sometimes heredity and gravity combine to create sagging, baggy eyebrows that not only make you look tired but also push downward on the eyelid and impede vision.

"For this problem I'd do a browlift," says Dr. Stegman. "A simple browlift can be done under local anesthesia in

the office or on an outpatient basis at a hospital. The incision is made right at the eyebrow or above it. We then remove some of the loose skin and suture.

"The incision will leave a scar," Dr. Stegman adds, "and it's best if you have good eyebrows to hide it. But often a browlift is all that's needed to give a patient better looks and better vision."

There's also a variation called a coronal browlift, which involves more extensive surgery. Unlike the other procedures, it must be done in a hospital under general anesthesia.

"The incision for a coronal browlift is made like a headband; it goes from ear to ear over the top of your head, about ¾ inch into the hairline. The scar is well hidden in the hairline, but the procedure can sometimes result in what I think of as a surprised look that isn't very natural," says Dr. Stegman.

Some Things to Consider

As in any surgical procedure, there are some risks in cosmetic dermatologic surgery. There is the possibility of infection or visible scarring, although for most patients the scar is barely visible and is hidden in the hairline or the fold of the eye. "You can have persistent redness in the scar or a slight unevenness where the doctor didn't remove the fat equally. These problems can be corrected, but they're problems nonetheless," cautions Dr. Stegman.

Since so much depends on the surgeon, it's important to spend the time to find the right one. Here are some guidelines from Dr. Stegman. "Ask for recommendations from friends who've had good results. Also, you can contact either the American Society for Dermatologic Surgery (312-869-3954), the American Academy of Facial Plastic and Reconstructive Surgery (1-800-332-FACE), the American Academy of Cosmetic Surgery (1-800-221-9808), or your local medical society for recommendations. It's your money and your face, so check several sources.

"When you consult with the doctor you've chosen, notice whether he or she is listening to your concerns. Is the doctor looking closely at you? Is he or she addressing your

problem and explaining what he or she feels is best for you?

"Look at pictures, but bear in mind the doctor is only going to show you good ones," says Dr. Stegman. "It's better to talk to a satisfied patient. Feel free to ask the doctor whether this is a procedure that he or she specializes in. Some dermatologic surgeons do mostly scalp transplants and little eye work or vice versa. If you're not comfortable with a doctor for whatever reason, find another one.

"Most important, no one should be talked into cosmetic surgery by either friends or a doctor."

PART IX: CHILDREN'S HEALTH NEWSFRONT

CHAPTER 34

When Food Becomes a Foe

Some good advice, from uncovering food foes to handling serious slip-ups.

For most kids, food sustains and nurtures the body. But for fifth-grader Michelle Bean, foods were foes. At 10 years old, Michelle was hospitalized with severe eczema, a staph infection, and asthma. Her weight hovered at 49 pounds, and her hair fell out. Her food allergies were so numerous that they read like a grocery list: milk, eggs, wheat, soy, corn, fish, cola.

Today, however, 18-year-old Michelle is a healthy nursing student. She can lunch with friends in the college cafeteria or sip Coke at the local pizza shop with no fear of ill effects. Her food allergies are gone—except for one: a lingering sensitivity to perch.

Michelle's story offers hope to parents of kids with food allergies—whether "mild" or "severe." Let's face it: Any food allergy is a handicap. It means juggled meals with the family. It can mean missed birthday parties or sleep-overs with friends—simply because you can't be sure what foods will be served. It can mean forfeiting everyday treats in

exchange for blander, less tasty food. Day after day, month after month, year after year, it's no fun to have to say no to foods you like. It's no wonder that parents—and kids—pray for the allergies to vanish.

What triggered Michelle Bean's turnaround? The credit belongs to controlled "food challenges" by an allergist and a carefully designed diet that enabled Michelle's immune system to outgrow its food hypersensitivities. And that's the news allergy specialists are trumpeting to parents of the thousands of children with adverse food reactions: Given the right medical treatment, *kids will outgrow most food allergies* (sometimes in a matter of months). But they will need plenty of support from Mom, Dad, and the rest of the family.

The Many Faces of Food Allergies

Today's news is encouraging, considering the fact that getting a handle on food allergies has never been easy. For one thing, experts aren't sure exactly how many kids suffer from food-related problems. Current research suggests that the number of children who have adverse food reactions is small—perhaps 4 to 6 percent of infants and 2 to 3 percent of older children. True food allergies represent only a small portion of these.

"A true food allergy or hypersensitivity (they're synonymous) is an immunologic reaction resulting from the ingestion of a food or food additive," explains Dean D. Metcalfe, M.D., of the National Institutes of Health in Bethesda, Maryland, who is head of the Adverse Reactions to Food Committee of the American Academy of Allergy and Immunology. "This reaction only occurs in some patients, and it may occur only after a small amount of the substance is ingested." (Some doctors refer to true allergies as "IgE mediated"—meaning that an antibody known as immunoglobulin E causes the allergic reaction when a certain food is eaten.)

A complication in corraling allergies is that your child's sensitivity may *not* be immunologic. A child can have a food intolerance—an abnormal physical response to a

food or food additive—such as a lactose intolerance. Children can be sensitive to certain chemicals, among them tartrazine (a yellow coloring used in foods and medicines) or sulfite (used to preserve foods and wines). Finally, adverse reactions are often caused by food poisoning—improperly prepared or contaminated food.

It would be easier to pinpoint allergic offenders if reactions were distinct. Alas, allergies can hide behind numerous masks, making it difficult to train the periscope on the offender. Food hypersensitivity can manifest itself as eczema, hives, stomachaches, headaches, inability to put on weight, nasal congestion, asthma, nausea, diarrhea, or colic.

With all these variables, it's a wonder that doctors ever unmask food foes. That's why parents must join forces with pediatricians and allergists to investigate possible allergens thoroughly. Pinpointing allergies is a slow, test-by-test process. (See "Unmasking Food Foes" on page 228.) But once your child has been clinically tested, you will know with confidence the cause of his or her symptoms. And you'll be better prepared to grapple with it.

News from the Front

In the battle against food allergies, the really encouraging news comes from front-running studies specifically examining children's food allergies. S. Allan Bock, M.D., of the National Jewish Center for Immunology and Respiratory Medicine in Denver, recently completed a three-year study of 480 children. In following these kids from birth to three years of age, Dr. Bock discovered that 80 percent of adverse food reactions occurred in the first year of life. When the problem food was eliminated from the diet, the child usually outgrew his or her sensitivity to that food within nine months (*Pediatrics*).

Other researchers agree that time and food avoidance can help a child's immune system overcome its hypersensitivity. One of these researchers is Hugh A. Sampson, M.D., a pediatric immunologist/allergist at the Children's

(continued on page 231)

Unmasking Food Foes

Although kids tend to be allergic to six common foods—eggs, peanuts, milk, soy, fish, and wheat—*any* food can be the source of food hypersensitivity. And because kids eat so many combinations of foods in a day, unmasking the food offender can be a long, tedious affair, even for the likes of a Sherlock Holmes.

Allergy specialists have come up with a variety of methods for targeting the culprit. Your allergist may use some or all of them, depending upon how quickly the allergen can be located. Here's a list of the most-used techniques for uncovering the causes of adverse food reactions.

The Food Diary

Just about every doctor will ask you to create a food diary. If you suspect your child has a food-related problem, you might even start the diary before you visit the doctor's office.

The food diary records what your child eats and how he or she feels afterward. "This can be a spiral 3 × 5 notebook that you keep in a pocket or purse. Fill it in when you're on hold on the telephone or in a grocery line," says allergy specialist Joann Blessing-Moore, M.D. In this diary, she says, you write down:

1. Everything your child ate each day. Be very specific. Instead of writing "hamburger," write "beef burger with tomato ketchup, onion, lettuce, and pickle on a white-flour roll."
2. A list of symptoms your child experienced that day, and when they occurred. Did the hives start 5 minutes after Jack ate white bread? Or did it take an hour for symptoms to develop?
3. The day's "score." Ask your child to rate his or her day. Would he or she give it a ten for good, a five

for okay, or a three for poor? This is a great way of getting a snapshot of your child's feelings, which you can refer to later as you modify the diet.

"The diary does the detective work," says Dr. Blessing-Moore. It points to possible allergens or flags a sensitivity to chemical additives, a lactose intolerance, or reactions caused by eating foods that contain high levels of histamines. The latter three problems are not strictly food allergies, because they don't create an immunologic response. But they do create real problems for the child, which you and the allergist can then address with diet.

Skin-Prick Tests and RAST Tests

Skin-prick tests (in which a small amount of a suspected allergen is placed under the skin), and radioallergosorbent, or RAST, tests (which measure the amount of an allergy-provoking antibody called IgE in the blood) are sometimes used to narrow the field: If your child doesn't react to a substance, he or she is not allergic to it. However, experts today don't consider these tests very reliable, for they can indicate an allergy where one does not exist. One youngster tested positive to 27 foods; further testing proved an allergy to 3. A restrictive diet should not be based solely on results from skin-prick or RAST tests.

The Elimination Diet

If the food diary or skin tests point to one or two offending foods, your pediatrician or allergist might try eliminating that food from your child's diet for a few weeks. Then the suspect foods are reintroduced one at a time. If an obvious reaction occurs—voilà! You've found the culprit. And that's sufficient evidence for your child to stay off that food for a period of time and be retested later, says pediatric allergist Hugh A. Sampson, M.D.

(continued)

Unmasking Food Foes—Continued

The elimination diet often works hand-in-glove with blind testing, especially if a child is supposedly allergic to a number of foods. "If you took somebody off four things—like milk, eggs, wheat, and soy—and their allergic symptoms went totally away, you'd still have to go on and do more workup, because that's a terrible diet to try to keep somebody on," says Dr. Sampson. You must be absolutely sure all four allergies exist before putting your child on such a nutritionally rigorous meal plan.

Single- and Double-Blind Testing

These are the most accurate but time-consuming food allergy testing methods, entailing frequent visits to the allergist's office or even an overnight stay in the hospital. Single-blind testing means your child may get a dose of a suspected allergen or a placebo (harmless blank substance). Your child doesn't know which he or she is getting, but the doctor does. Double-blind testing means your child and the person administering the dose don't know whether a placebo or an allergen is being given. These methods achieve objective results, since any reaction that occurs is most likely a reaction to the actual food rather than an "expected" reaction to a food that is only suspected of being an allergen.

Blind testing food allows the doctor to determine whether the substance really does create an allergic reaction and, if so, what sort of reaction results. It lets you separate the foods you *think* create a problem from those that actually do.

The Food Challenge

Children who have abstained from eating an offending food for a period of time (perhaps three months to a year) should be rechallenged at intervals. Since kids

can outgrow many allergies, the challenge is needed to see if the allergy still exists.

Blind testing is often used as the food rechallenge. In some cases, where true allergy seems unlikely, the reintroduction of food can be done at home.

Note: Food trials should be done under a doctor's supervision. Generally, that means reintroduction in the doctor's office. Many parents in the past have done some testing themselves, and they freely admit their difficulty in interpreting the results. Experts also worry about a severe life-threatening reaction that might occur far from medical help. In the same vein, diets that suggest you go on some kind of food elimination plan and then reintroduce food on your own at home should only be done with a physician's approval and where the condition is non-life-threatening—for example, a food that just gives your child very mild problems like a stuffy nose. But if you think that hives or asthma are due to food, the reintroduction of foods believed to be culprits should be done only with extreme caution and under the guidance of a physician.

Medical and Surgical Center of the Johns Hopkins University School of Medicine in Baltimore. "Our studies suggest that a child's chances of losing a food allergy are much better if he or she goes completely off the food for a finite period of time than if he or she keeps getting low quantities," says Dr. Sampson. In some cases, the allergy disappears in a matter of a year or two.

To determine whether an allergy has been outgrown, Dr. Sampson "rechallenges" the child once a year with blind testing. (See "Unmasking Food Foes" on page 228 for more information on this testing method.) If the test food no longer gives the child a problem, it's deemed safe to reintroduce into the diet. In the case of Michelle Bean, these annual challenges mapped out her body's progress in overcoming her hypersensitivities.

Farewell, Foul Food

Abstinence also seems to be the best way to handle food problems that are not classified as true allergies. "As an overall concept, anything that you would react to adversely in foods is best handled by avoidance," says Dr. Metcalfe. Whether your child is bothered by spinach or by sulfites, say farewell to the food and you banish the debilitating side effects. This is especially true for those allergies that aren't outgrown, such as the allergy to peanuts or shellfish. In these cases, abstinence is essential, because reactions can get worse with each ingestion.

Children's food sensitivities are, on the whole, different from those of adults. "Eighty-five percent of the reactions of children in the 3-month to 20-year range occur with eggs, peanuts, milk, soy, fish, and wheat," says Dr. Sampson. "Kids react to lots of other things, too—like rice, potatoes, pork, and bananas—but it's not as frequent." Infants are often irritated by fruit juices and milk. These problems usually disappear as the infant's digestive system matures. In contrast, adults tend to be hypersensitive to tree nuts, peanuts, eggs, fish, and shellfish such as lobster, shrimp, and crab.

The Real Issue—Nutrition

"We may be dealing with food intolerance, but what we're really talking about is good nutrition," asserts Joann Blessing-Moore, M.D., an allergic/immunologic/pediatric pulmonologist at the Palo Alto Medical Clinic and a member of the clinical faculty at Stanford University in Palo Alto, California.

"It's important to treat allergies early and treat them aggressively," she adds. Part of that aggressive treatment is a sound nutritional plan, one that is sympathetic to a child's feelings.

"It's not easy at any age to cope with a special diet," says Dr. Blessing-Moore. "It's hard for kids to speak up at restaurants, at birthday parties, or at milk time in kindergarten. Even adults who have food allergies will often ask

themselves, 'Should I make a big deal of this?' when eating in public."

"A lot of this is harder for the mother than the child," says Deborah Duguid of Jacksonville, Florida, whose six-year-old daughter Cassie is allergic to milk, eggs, and peanuts. "But as the child gets older, it's also hard for her. Now that Cassie is going to school, she's becoming aware of some of her limitations. Before, she never knew what cookies or cupcakes were, because she'd never had them."

If your son is allergic to chocolate, his diet won't suffer from its absence (although his sweet tooth might). But if you must scratch a more fundamental food off the menu, it's more difficult to ensure nutritional adequacy.

"Even if you do something as simple as take milk out of a child's diet, you have to be *very* careful that that child gets an adequate supply of calcium," says Dr. Metcalfe. "The decision to alter diet should only be done with great caution."

Never take your child off a number of foods without being absolutely sure that those foods are actually the source of problems. Few tykes or teenagers have more than two actual allergies. "We've found that even though some of our children may have large numbers of positive skin tests, 80 percent react to only one or two foods," says Dr. Sampson.

When a child has severe food allergies, a dietitian's assistance is invaluable in planning well-rounded meals. "One of the concerns with children who have allergies is that if you combine the foods a child can't tolerate with foods that he or she doesn't like, plus any foods the parents *think* the child can't tolerate, you can get a very limited diet," says L. Kathleen Mahan, a registered dietitian who is a consulting nutritionist in private practice in Seattle and coauthor of *Food, Nutrition and Diet Therapy.*

Mahan asks her patients to keep food diaries, which she evaluates with a computer. "Our computer analysis gives parents pretty accurate information," she says. It points out which foods a child should be eating to improve his or her diet. If those foods can't be worked in, then supplements are recommended. "But at least our supplementa-

tion is focused, because we know why we're adding things to the diet," says Mahan.

How can you create a varied, balanced, and wholesome diet for your food-sensitive child? The experts offer these tips for allergy-free meals.

Know your labels. "In this country, we are really fortunate that food is labeled the way it is," Mahan states. The careful parent can scrutinize the ingredients list on prepackaged food for offending substances. The trouble is, manufacturers often use cryptic terms—like "albumin" for egg—which you must become familiar with. (See "The Shopping Safari" on page 236 for help in cracking food-label "codes.")

Reading labels will initially triple your time in the grocery store. But with experience and persistence, you'll gain a repertoire of products that you can trust. Remember, however, that manufacturers sometimes change ingredients, especially in baked goods. Your best defense is to review the label of even your most favored brand every few months.

Start simple. You'll inevitably find yourself in the kitchen making more meals from scratch, because that's the easiest way to be sure the food is allergen free. "In the beginning, it'll help if you avoid eating out," says Mahan. "I also recommend that you start with simple foods, just so you get used to the diet, begin to see your child's symptoms improve, and feel a sense of accomplishment."

Many parents recommend compiling a scrapbook of basic recipes. Children with egg, milk, and wheat allergies (the three most common) require a basic bread recipe, a basic cookie recipe, a sweet bread recipe—like banana bread—and a cracker recipe. "Once you get those four things down, that makes meals a lot easier," Mahan states.

Find new foods. Scout the ethnic or health food markets for new foods that can pinch-hit for ones your child can't eat. A little curiosity can take you a long way. Rosanne Patten, of Schnectady, New York, was determined to indulge her young son Benjamin in the traditional, messy, but enjoyable childhood experience of spaghetti and meatballs. But Ben was allergic to milk, eggs, wheat, beef, corn, and soy. So Rosanne found rice noodles in a Japanese

restaurant and made little lamb meatballs. The meal was a splendidly sloppy success. There are other practical hints from the experts, too:

- Soy milk that comes in a brick pack with a straw is perfect for school snack time for the milk-sensitive child.
- Corn oil and soy oil are safe to use even if your child is allergic to corn or soy. The reason: The allergens have been removed in processing.

Cookbooks for people with food allergies often discuss substitute foods—and some even offer microwave recipes. (See "Recommended Recipe Reading" on page 241 and "The Shopping Safari" on page 236 for more diet tips.)

Plan a bag-lunch strategy. It's easier all the way around to have your son or daughter pack a school lunch. You have more control over what he or she eats. Remember to provide substitute treats so your child doesn't feel like he or she is being punished. One mother of an allergic kindergartener leaves a bag of her daughter's snack at school so she won't be left out at milk time.

Make main meals a family affair. Should you completely change the family's eating habits to accommodate a child with one or two food sensitivities, such as peanuts or soy? It's not necessary, says Dr. Metcalfe, because in most cases, removing a few food items doesn't alter the family's diet greatly. You may like preparing individual portions (which may be necessary when the sensitivity includes wheat, eggs, and milk), or you may find it easier if dishes do double duty.

But be aware, says Mahan, that "when food allergy management is done most effectively, the whole family's diet changes somewhat. Certainly you can make the allergic child's lunch sandwich different from his or her brother's or sister's. But when the child who has the allergy can also eat the major meal, you have the best compliance."

If you don't make it a family affair, someone ends up being the "gatekeeper," whose job it is to keep the allergic child from eating offensive foods. The gatekeeper is usually one of the parents—and it's an unpleasant position. "It's easier to make a bean and rice dish or a meat and a

(continued on page 240)

The Shopping Safari: Hunting through Labels for Allergy-Free Foods

Few people have the time to make every morsel of their allergic child's diet from scratch. So they turn to frozen, canned, or baked goods to form part of their child's meals. Selecting only "safe foods" is essential—and that's where label-reading skills come into action.

Ingredient labels alert you to foods that will antagonize your child. But there's a catch: You have to know the terms food manufacturers employ on these listings. For instance, are you aware that "albumin" means egg whites, and that "caseinate" means milk? Ignorance can lead to disastrous mistakes, slip-ups that no parent wants to make.

The following material was developed by Hugh A. Sampson, M.D., of the Johns Hopkins University School of Medicine, while he was at Duke University Medical Center's Department of Pediatrics; it is reprinted and adapted here with his permission. It will alert you to the "key words" that must be avoided, as well as offering some diet tips. Armed with this label-reading savvy and the hunter's eye, you can effectively stalk the grocery shelves for your child's allergy-free foods.

Egg-Restricted Diet

You may not use even small amounts of egg in any recipe. Learn to look for "egg words" on the labels of the foods you buy. Avoid any food that has even *one* of these foods listed as an ingredient:

- Egg.
- Egg white.
- Dried egg.
- Albumin.

Note that different brands of the same food may contain different ingredients. Also, food producers sometimes change their ingredients.

Diet tips: (1) When baking, substitute ½ teaspoon baking powder and ½ tablespoon vinegar for each egg omitted; (2) Egg replacers are allowed, such as Golden Harvest or Ener-G egg replacers; (3) Delicatessens, large groceries, or health food stores are sources for eggless mayonnaise, eggless pancake mix, and corn noodles without egg; (4) Try using one of the following as a "binder" in your egg-free baked goods: tahini (ground sesame seeds)—2 tablespoons per egg; any nut butter—2 tablespoons per egg; oat flour—2 tablespoons plus 1 tablespoon water per egg.

Milk-Restricted Diet

You may not use even small amounts of any milk product in the diet. Learn to look for "milk words" on the label. Avoid any food that has even one of these words listed as an ingredient:

- Milk.
- Whey.
- Calcium caseinate.
- Butter.
- Dried milk solids.
- Cheese.
- Casein.
- Margarine.
- Sodium caseinate.
- Curds.

Note that different brands of the same food may contain different ingredients. Also, food companies periodically change the ingredients in their products.

Diet tips: (1) Kosher milk-free foods are labeled "parve" or "pareve." They may be found in Jewish delicatessens or in large grocery stores. Look for

(continued)

The Shopping Safari—Continued
breads, margarines, and processed meats with this word. (2) Use milk-free margarine and substitute soy formula/water/juice for liquid in baking. (3) Use Coffee Rich or fruit juice on cereal. (4) Salt-free margarines are often milk-free. Check the label.

Soy-Restricted Diet
You may not even use a small amount of any soy protein-containing food. Soy is found in many forms and is present in many processed foods. You must learn to read all food labels for "soy words." Avoid any food that has even one of these words listed as an ingredient:

- Soybean.
- Soy flour.
- Soy protein.
- Soy protein isolate.
- Tamari.
- Soya.
- Soy.
- Vegetable broth (unless other source of vegetable is noted).
- Cereal (unless other source of cereal is noted).
- Vegetable protein (unless other source of vegetable is noted).

On the other hand, *some soy by-products are allowed.* The reason for this is that the allergenic, protein portion of soy has been removed in processing. So carefully check labels for the following soy words. These soy products may be eaten.

- Soy oil/soybean oil.
- Lecithin/soy lecithin.
- Hydrolyzed soy protein (also listed as hydrolyzed vegetable protein or hydrolyzed plant protein).

Note that food companies frequently change the ingredients in their products.

Wheat-Restricted Diet

You may not use even a small amount of any wheat product in the diet. Again, you must learn to read all food labels for "wheat words." Avoid any food that has even one of these words listed as an ingredient:

- Wheat.
- Graham flour.
- Flour.
- Farina.
- Wheat germ.
- Semolina.
- Wheat starch.
- Bran (may be eaten if it's listed as corn bran, oat bran, etc.).
- Modified food starch (may be eaten if the source food is listed, such as "modified food starch, from corn").

Note that food companies frequently change the ingredients in their products. This is especially true in baked goods. You must always read the labels.

Diet tips: (1) To make an all-purpose flour without wheat, mix 1 cup cornstarch, 2 cups rice flour, 2 cups soy flour, and 3 cups potato starch flour. Use equal cups of this mixture to replace wheat flour in recipes. Bake at lower temperature for a longer period of time. The finished product will be crustier. (2) Here are figures for flour exchange: 1 cup wheat flour equals 1 ⅓ cup oat flour or 1¼ cups rye flour or ⅝ cup potato starch flour or ⅞ cup rice flour or ½ cup barley flour or ¾ cup cornmeal (coarse). (3) For thickening exchange: 1 tablespoon wheat flour equals ½ tablespoon cornstarch or ½ tablespoon potato starch flour or 2 teaspoons quick tapioca. (4) Crush rice cereal to make breading crumbs.

rice dish—something the whole family can have," Mahan says. "But you know, that applies to management of any chronic disorder in which diet is important. When I work with children who are overweight, I get my best results when the entire family changes their eating and cooking habits."

Handling the Occasional Lapse

Most of the time, even the youngest of kids won't eat stuff that they know makes them feel terrible. By carefully explaining to your child what foods make him or her ill, you educate the child to question strange foods and to avoid things that might cause a reaction. "Many of my little patients know *a lot* about their food allergies," says Dr. Blessing-Moore. Dr. Sampson trained his allergic daughter, at age 2½, to ask if a food had eggs or to say "I can't eat eggs."

But every now and then, nature throws a curve ball. Maybe a friend or sibling hands your son a problem food and says it's okay to eat. Or maybe those cupcakes are just too tempting for your daughter to resist. Dr. Sampson recalls how his daughter one day out of the blue told a babysitter, "I want eggs!" And even parents slip and forget to read a label before serving a generous helping of an offending food. Because mistakes happen, you must have backup plans.

How do you treat a slip-up? "If reactions have always been eczema, and never anything else, and the child eats something that flares his or her eczema, then you treat the eczema like you usually treat it," says Dr. Metcalfe. Stuffy noses and such can be treated with benadryl or the medication your child normally uses.

But if your child is extremely sensitive to a food, extra caution is critical. "We all worry about those children who have reactions that are severe and may progress to be life-threatening—in other words, anaphylaxis," says Dr. Metcalfe. "In those cases, if the child makes a mistake and nothing happens, then there's nothing you have to do. But

Recommended Recipe Reading

To help parents with allergic children in the search for substitute foods and recipes, the following books are recommended.

The Allergy Gourmet, The Allergy Baker, The Allergy Cookie Jar, and *The Allergy Chef,* all by Carol Rudoff (available from the Allergy Publications Group of the American Allergy Association, Menlo Park, California).

Caring and Cooking for the Allergic Child, by Linda L. Thomas (published by Sterling Publishing Company, New York).

The Allergy Guide to Brand-Name Foods and Food Additives, by Stephanie Bernardo Johns (published by the New American Library/Plume Books, New York and Scarborough, Ontario).

if he or she has a severe reaction, then you must be prepared to treat that reaction *immediately.*"

And that means treating it with epinephrine, a form of adrenaline, that is available in small, self-dispensing kits. If your child is at home, you'll do the injection. If your child is at school or day care or Sunday school, another adult must be prepared to administer treatment swiftly. Older kids can be taught to inject themselves—and they should carry the kits with them any time they'll be eating out.

Because anaphylaxis is so extreme—sometimes leading to death—extra precaution must be taken to avoid any contact with the troublesome food. School children who have had anaphylactoid reactions in the past will often stay out of the school cafeteria if the food is being served that day.

Life-threatening allergies are less common, advises Dr. Metcalfe. Most parents of allergic patients, while they need

The Behavioral Debate

Can food allergies affect the way your child behaves? Yes and no, say the experts.

"It's certainly true that if a child is having allergies, the asthma or hives or abdominal discomfort is going to interrupt his or her ability to concentrate. The child won't behave normally," says Dean D. Metcalfe, M.D., of the National Institutes of Health.

"It's like any person who's sick; behavior is different," agrees Hugh A. Sampson, M.D.

"And if those children use medicines, their behavior will also be altered," Dr. Metcalfe adds. "An ephedrine kind of compound will make them nervous or jittery. An antihistamine may make them sleepy. This is one of the problems that allergists face in structuring medications for children in school. You want to get something that doesn't affect their ability to perform."

The behavioral debate hinges on statements that very mild, subclinical allergies—ones that have no obvious clinical effects like asthma or hives or abdominal pain—can lead to behavioral problems, and on statements that hyperactivity can be the sole manifestation of a food allergy. To date, however, no

to know about the possibility of severe reactions, will not need to worry that their child will react in this way. Kids generally experience mild or manageable reactions and handle them with good humor. Mom and Dad often suffer the most—from guilt, when a suspect food has inadvertently been introduced into the diet. Dr. Blessing-Moore sees that as the wrong attitude to take.

"You don't want kids to get paranoid about eating," she says. "So don't be critical of a slip-up. Use it as a positive thing: You've just given your child a food rechallenge! And rechallenges are essential in determining whether an allergy has been outgrown."

clinical studies have backed these claims. Parents and doctors ought to examine all options before claiming that food is creating behavioral difficulties.

"This is a profound problem," stresses Dr. Metcalfe, "because if that child's hyperactivity is due to something else—for example, inattention at home, poor dietary habits, another illness not being properly treated, problems with other children at school, or poor vision—and you attribute it to corn hypersensitivity, you're doing that child a *great* disservice."

If you're convinced your child has allergy-related behavioral problems and you want to find out for sure, Dr. Metcalfe strongly advises that you go to a doctor who's willing to do blind testing and follow your child's progress.

"In other words, you can explore that hypothesis. But you *can't* do it by announcing, 'Let's take corn out of the diet and feed the child these foods and see if it affects his or her behavior.' " Why? Because, as any researcher knows, just the fact that you're giving the child more attention will modify his or her behavior—but it won't be a long-term change. The better route is to work with a good allergist to unearth the real cause. You and your child will be much happier in the long run.

The key is to have a balanced view of allergies. Don't let them throw you into a panic, but don't get complacent, either. "Sometimes you can get away with eating a little of the food; then you start hoping you're no longer sensitive; then you get casual about it," Dr. Metcalfe notes. "As a rule, these problems should be taken very, very seriously." Wait until your child gets a clean bill of health from your allergist before letting him or her dip into the once-forbidden larder.

Parents of kids with food hypersensitivities all talk of their "it'll never end" feelings. They vividly recall the exhausting complications of juggling a limited diet. When

you're facing a day like that, be positive and consistent. Remember, the chances of your child outgrowing allergies are great if you persist with the careful diet. Says Deborah Duguid: "It's important to be firm and not to give in when the child is begging for a food or when you're tired and don't feel like making a separate meal."

And think how good your child will feel once the allergies disappear. As one mother said of her daughter's ecstatic introduction to ketchup: "She thought she'd died and gone to heaven." Those are moments of jubilation that your persistence, care, and support today will make possible tomorrow.

CHAPTER 35

Modern Management of Childhood Asthma

Putting childhood asthma in its place is like putting an ailing business back on its feet: Good management is the key.

Michele Urban knew something was wrong when she checked on her infant daughter one day in 1983.

"I leaned over her bassinet while she was sleeping and heard her wheeze. I could tell she was having distress," says Urban, who with her husband, son, and daughter lives in the western Pennsylvania town of Latrobe.

Thus began the first of two dozen hospital visits for a blonde, hazel-eyed little girl named Jayme. She learned to walk in the hospital and celebrated her first three birthdays there. She got a trip in an ambulance with an intravenous

tube strapped to her arm and once frightened her family by beginning to turn blue.

Along with nearly 3 million other Americans under age 18, Jayme has asthma, the most prevalent chronic illness of childhood.

But while people once looked at asthma with the dread of a life sentence, the news about asthma is actually bright. While not curable, even severe asthma is controllable. Careful treatment and medication are so effective in preventing or squelching flare-ups that several athletes have managed asthma all the way to Olympic competition.

Consider 4-year-old Jayme Urban. After treatment at the Pittsburgh Rehabilitation Institute to bring her case under control, she came home to a new life. Her medication was simplified and her bedroom moved away from the pollen-rich garden side of the house. Where once she couldn't toddle across the room without wheezing, today she goes to gymnastics class and ballet.

Jayme's case is severe, but asthma can also be so mild it goes undiagnosed. It's a disease that defies neat labels. There is no tidy statistic to show its full cost, but clearly it's enormous. One mother estimates prescription medicine for her boys, one mildly and the other moderately asthmatic, costs $325 a month. Add to that $60 in monthly electric bills for running an air filter in her home.

And the price in quality of living can be high. "Having a sick child can wreak havoc on a family," says another parent. "It can be very difficult on a marriage." Nighttime flare-ups make the hours of lost sleep beyond counting.

Children sometimes pay in the currency of academic performance. Asthma ranks as the leading cause of school absences, with at least 20 percent of missed days attributed to it. That's another reason why learning how to manage the disease is so important.

Anatomy of an Asthma Attack

Asthma's trademark is narrowing of the airways. It can make the ordinarily effortless business of breathing a struggle, leaving children pale, perspiring, and exhausted.

"As they get sicker, you can see they're working harder to breathe," says David Murphy, M.D., head of pulmonology at Deborah Heart and Lung Center in Browns Mills, New Jersey.

The windpipe is the portal of entry for every breath. It divides into two main airways or bronchi, which branch treelike into an ever-smaller network deep in the lungs. Asthma tightens these airway muscles in what physicians call bronchospasm. It also inflames the sensitive inner mucous membrane, causing swelling, and spurs mucus glands into overdrive.

Constriction, swelling, excess mucus: All obstruct air passages, making it difficult to fully exhale stale air and draw in fresh.

Wheezing or whistling sounds, from vibrations as exhaled air rushes through obstructed bronchi, are classic symptoms. But attacks have many signs: constant coughing or throat-clearing to expel mucus, vomiting, increased breathing rate, restlessness, and hunched posture, as extra muscles join the effort to breathe.

It gets scary.

"We were traveling to Atlanta to catch a plane. All of a sudden he started having an attack," recalls one mother of an experience with her son, who was then in kindergarten.

"I knew it was severe. He coughed and coughed until finally he threw up. He needed medicine. So I'm in the back seat of this rental car on a lonely interstate, my child throwing up in my lap. My husband was driving, saying 'What should I do?'

"I was always proud of being able to keep a calm exterior to present to my son. But on the interstate that night, I just screamed, 'Take the next exit!' And at the exit there was a sign from God: a hospital sign with a blue arrow."

Pulling Asthma's Trigger

Asthma attacks can develop quickly, like this one, or gradually. "Triggers," the things that set off attacks, are complex and not fully understood. Many children react to several different things, and even when physicians begin to

understand the dynamics of a given case, the triggers can change.

Identifying what sets off asthma takes time. Physicians often suggest keeping an activity-and-medication diary to spot patterns in the following areas.

Allergies. An estimated 80 percent of childhood asthma cases are related to allergies, reactions produced by the immune system.

When foreign materials like pollen or viruses contact the body, certain cells go to the body's defense with antibodies to neutralize the visitors. In an allergic reaction, however, one kind of antibody becomes part of the problem by triggering the release of chemicals (histamine is probably the most familiar) that in vulnerable children cause asthma to flare.

The list of potential allergens—plant pollens, animal dander, molds—seems endless. Dust balls, where tiny house mites can share living quarters with any or all of the above, are allergy factories.

Experts discourage moving to a different part of the country to avoid allergies. Improvement is often only temporary, and there is always the possibility of trading the old allergy for a new one. But good housekeeping and avoidance of known problems is recommended. A first-grader sensitive to furry creatures shouldn't get a desk next to the class's pet gerbil.

Physicians sometimes initiate allergy tests and treatment with shots to reduce sensitivity to unavoidable allergens.

Irritants. A number of substances, such as smoke, perfume, and aerosol sprays, can provoke flare-ups. They appear to irritate the upper airways but are not considered allergens because they do not involve the chemical reaction of allergies.

Infections. Upper respiratory infections, especially viruses, can cause asthma symptoms.

Exercise. Experts recognize, but cannot entirely explain, exercise as a trigger. But that's not to say that being a couch potato is therapeutic. Exercise with appropriate medication is a vital component of treatment, even in severe cases. It should be undertaken only with the advice and guidance of a doctor, however.

The grab bag. Various other substances—air pollutants and certain food additives (such as sulfites), for example—appear to precipitate some children's asthma.

Emotions. Even emotions can trigger attacks in children who have asthma. Anger, fear, and stress can all be culprits. The American Lung Association cites the case of a teenager who, when away from home, would have an attack when she realized she had forgotten her medication. Emotions can also translate into counter-productive behavior, such as skipping medicine or smoking cigarettes.

Keeping Asthma under Control

Today's better understanding of asthma makes it something careful management generally can control, instead of a disability that catapults patients from one attack to the next.

One important element of good management is medication—the right medicine at the right time. It may sound simple, but it's not. There are many different medicines that do different things, some with potential side effects that have an impact on a child's health, school life, and self-image.

Even *taking* medicine—in bead-filled capsules, tablets, liquids, inhaled mists, and powder—gets complicated. And because a child's symptoms are likely to change over time, medication often requires periodic fine-tuning. Parents who've traveled this road frequently offer the same advice: *Find a good physician.* That means one who explains things clearly, stays up to date, and makes adjustments in medication as needed. (See "The Asthma Medicine Chest" on page 249 for information on drugs, their uses, and side effects.)

Exercising Good Management

Something else doctors prescribe, with quite positive side effects, is exercise.

"If you're in top form, even if you're still asthmatic,

(continued on page 252)

The Asthma Medicine Chest

There are so many drugs currently used to treat children with asthma that confusion's almost impossible to avoid. It's easier to keep track of them if you think of them as falling into four broad groups.

Theophylline

You may already have heard of theophylline, the most widely prescribed asthma medication in the United States and one considered quite effective. It is a "bronchodilator," which means it relaxes the muscles around the airways to reverse obstruction. It comes in many forms, including sustained-release preparations that reduce the frequency of doses so children and parents can get a full night's sleep.

Physicians note that it can make some kids jumpy, especially when first prescribed. "I often said that the doctor ought to prescribe Valium for the mother at the same time that he prescribed the medicine for the child," quips one parent.

Recent research has raised the issue of subtle behavioral effects in school. In one study of 20 kids aged 6 to 12, teachers were able to pick out the children on high-dose sustained-release theophylline, noting their distracted behavior.

The researchers, from the University of California at Los Angeles, say their findings underscore the importance of vigilance on the part of parents, teachers, and physicians supervising children on these medicines (*Pediatrics*).

Because establishing the correct dosage is important—too much can cause side effects—physicians often do tests to check blood theophylline levels.

(continued)

The Asthma Medicine Chest—Continued

Other Bronchodilators

These go by various names—adrenergic drugs, sympathomimetics, beta-agonists, adrenalinlike drugs—and come in a number of preparations, usually to be swallowed or inhaled. They are used to treat and prevent flare-ups.

Inhalation has the advantage of putting the medicine right on target, enhancing effectiveness and reducing side effects. The disadvantages? Inhalation can be tricky, especially for younger children. Physicians also warn that, to avoid overdoses, patients must adhere to prescribed amounts with an inhaler just as with medicines taken by pill or spoon.

Don't hesitate to ask questions if you are uncertain of your physician's instructions. Pharmaceutical companies and inventive doctors have developed several devices and techniques to help patients master inhalation.

Cromolyn

This drug (brand name, Intal) is used to *prevent* flare-ups and is believed to be free of side effects.

"Of the newer drugs that are available, I think cromolyn is one of the important ones," says Hunter Smith, M.D., of the National Jewish Center for Immunology and Respiratory Medicine, a Denver institute that treats asthma patients from across the country. "Cromolyn is excellent in preventing exercise-induced asthma and useful in lowering steroid doses," he says.

Researchers believe the medicine, which patients usually inhale, blocks the allergic reaction.

It does have disadvantages, though, and important differences from other asthma medicines. First, it's preventive and does not treat an attack in progress. Second, most often it must be used regularly, and it

takes time before becoming effective. Doctors also say it's expensive.

Steroids

Physicians find steroids very effective in helping children with severe asthma and in reversing attacks. But they also worry about serious potential side effects with long-term oral use, including interference with normal growth. Long-term use can also redistribute body fat, notes Dr. Smith. It can cause unflattering changes in appearance—a puffy, round face or "buffalo hump" of fat at the back of the neck—at a time for kids when appearance is everything.

In deciding on long-term use of steroids, the problems imposed by asthma have to be weighed against the potential side effects of the drug. There are several ways to minimize side effects, however. Oral steroids are usually prescribed in short, diminishing "bursts." Also, inhaled steroids, an innovation of the 1970s, and steroid nasal sprays act directly on the site of the problem and have less effect on the rest of the body.

Steroids used for asthma are a synthetic version of a natural hormone. They are not the same as anabolic steroids used by body builders.

Better Drugs on the Way

New medicines offer kids with asthma even more hope for a bright future. Researchers are very optimistic about a synthetic agent called ketotifen. It is believed to stabilize the cells involved in allergic reactions. It's administered orally to patients as a preventive medication.

Although the drug is now being tested in medical centers throughout the country, it has been marketed abroad for about five years, according to the New Jersey pharmaceutical firm that hopes to market it here.

you're better off," says Bea Maier, Ph.D., program coordinator of the asthma program at the Rehabilitation Institute of Pittsburgh, where severely asthmatic children can get treatment and attend school at the institute during stays of two months to a year. "Young patients usually are in poor shape when they arrive at the institute," says Dr. Maier. "They've missed out on school sports, gained weight on steroid treatment, and become accustomed to inactivity." Establishing a simple, effective medication regimen that minimizes steroids, improving fitness, and addressing emotional problems are key treatment goals in the program.

The same thinking applies at the National Jewish Center for Immunology and Respiratory Medicine, in Denver. "Many of our patients are on steroids," says Hunter Smith, M.D. "Steroids have a negative impact on bone and muscle tissue, and exercise helps counter that."

Hospitalization at these institutions isn't just to stabilize a child's asthma. It's to teach families how to take charge of asthma so the patient won't be back.

"That's one of the most important things—teaching the child and the family how to handle fluctuations and the importance of early treatment—to convince patients that with proper care they can get better. They can become normal, or close to normal. But it takes a fair amount of cooperation with the medical regimen," says Dr. Smith.

Kids Monitor Symptoms

The teaching process can begin early—as early as preschool. Children can learn to describe how they feel and blow into a peak-flow meter (see "Going with the Flow" on page 253), Dr. Maier says. They can become adept at knowing their symptoms and limits.

Since the 1970s, a proliferation of education programs aimed at asthma management education have emerged. One of the programs begins right in the emergency room with a slide show. Physicians and therapists in many communities teach family seminars using their own or prepackaged formats. And studies evaluating these programs suggest that good ones can reduce repeat visits to the

emergency room and help families cope better.

In one study, researchers from the University of Michigan and Columbia University in New York City examined an education program to see if it really changed behavior. They found that youngsters who went through the program reported more use of productive coughing (to expel mucus), relaxation and breathing exercises, and staying calm to manage their asthma. Kids also reported feeling less worried about restrictions their asthma imposed (*Patient Education and Counseling*).

Experts believe that all of these things—expanding medical understanding of asthma, using medicines correctly, better-informed patients—make asthma a disease that can be controlled. But they warn against complacency.

Heading Off Trouble

Childhood deaths from asthma are rare. Figures from the National Center for Health Statistics for 1984 reflect 96

Going with the Flow

How do you know when a child's breathing difficulty has reached the danger point? Specialists recommend keeping a peak-flow meter on hand. It's a small, relatively inexpensive device that gives a glimpse of the degree of airway obstruction by measuring the peak rate of air forcibly exhaled.

It's not a new idea. Physicians a century ago asked patients to blow out candles for the same reason, according to one researcher.

Using a peak-flow meter can signal an impending attack even before a child feels it coming on, says Geisinger Medical Center's Diane Schuller, M.D. "When you live with a chronic condition for a long time, sometimes you can't remember what is normal." The meter gives an objective measurement of the situation.

deaths among youngsters under age 15, most of them elementary school age children. But researchers have noticed that when they gather fatality figures from the past 25 years and put them on a graph, the falling death rate of the late 1960s begins to climb in the late 1970s.

It's a paradox that troubles physicians, who at a number of hospitals have dug deep into case histories in a search for answers. Delays in seeking treatment and inadequate recognition of the seriousness of asthma are two explanations researchers have suggested.

Where Can I Get Help?

If you're a parent new to asthma, the veterans have some advice: Learn how to live with it. It will take more than medicine, says Nancy Sander, a Fairfax, Virginia, mother of four. It takes a way of life.

She knows. It took several years to bring her 9-year-old daughter's complex tangle of symptoms under control. Staying ahead of the asthma means starting her daughter on preventive medication six weeks before the family vacation. It means having a pocket-sized peak-flow meter on hand. It means knowing how to use a nebulizer for medicines to be inhaled.

It also means dealing with the practical problems that physicians may not tell you about. How do you prepare your asthmatic child to stay overnight with a friend? How do you keep your house "trigger-free" without being tyrannized by a Dust Buster?

Sander decided to pass along what she learned. And so, in a Virginia kitchen on a broken typewriter in 1985, a newsletter and a support system were born: Mothers of Asthmatics. It's one of many sources of information and support. A sampler of these sources is listed here.

- Mothers of Asthmatics, 5316 Summit Drive, Fairfax, VA 22030. The group's monthly newsletter for

One study done at the National Jewish Center for Immunology and Respiratory Medicine looked at 21 cases between 1973 and 1982 in which children had died during a severe attack after leaving the hospital, sometimes several years after leaving. Researchers compared these to cases of similarly ill children who were still living. They found that psychological factors set the fatalities apart from the others (*Journal of the American Medical Association*).

Child psychiatrist Bruce Miller, M.D., doing follow-up

parents of asthmatic and allergic children is $10 for 12 issues.

- Lung Line. Call 1-800-222-LUNG toll-free between 8:00 A.M. and 5:00 P.M. Mountain Time from anywhere in the contiguous 48 states (in Denver, call 355-LUNG). This hotline is sponsored by the National Jewish Center for Immunology and Respiratory Medicine in Denver. Specially trained nurses will answer general questions and refer callers to physicians who have served at the center as fellows. The hotline gets from 150 to 200 calls every business day, so be patient if you get a busy signal. Ask for the center's 20-page booklet, "Your Child and Asthma."
- Your local library. Much has been written on asthma. One good book is *Asthma: The Complete Guide to Self-Management of Asthma and Allergies for Patients and Their Families,* by Allan M. Weinstein, M.D. (McGraw-Hill, $17.95).
- Your local American Lung Association. It distributes literature and a package called "Superstuff" for parents and kids to use at home. Several local affiliates also sponsor patient-education classes. For further information and a copy of "Superstuff," contact your American Lung Association, listed in the white pages of the telephone book.

research at the National Jewish Center, believes that this underscores the importance of paying attention to psychological problems in kids with asthma, because risks appear greater for children engulfed in conflict. "I think children who are emotionally and behaviorally disturbed and unable to comply with a medical regimen are at great risk. I would say depression is one of the major forms of emotional disturbance related to untoward outcomes."

He cautions against minimizing or denying a child's feelings. "Parents and doctors need to be reminded to think about the child's feelings. You must address the psychological aspects, not deny them. We know asthma is not an illness that is curable. The key is to look positively on your life and make accommodations for dealing with it."

Breathing Easy at Summer Camp

Managing asthma is a way of life each August on 567 wooded acres along the Juniata River in Pennsylvania when Camp Breathe Easy moves in. Here, blowing in a peak-flow meter, a small gadget to check lung function, is *de rigueur.*

With grass and trees and campfires burning bright, this camp for asthmatic children is the antithesis of everything medical director Diane Schuller, M.D., normally preaches.

"I've been astonished that children in an environment quite hostile to allergy sufferers do exceptionally well," says Dr. Schuller, director of the Pediatric Allergy, Immunology, and Pulmonary Department at Geisinger Medical Center in central Pennsylvania.

"It's given me a tremendous appreciation of how well the medications work and of how important it is for children to come in early for treatment."

CHAPTER 36

Living with Juvenile Diabetes

Medical advances can almost guarantee a normal childhood, and the prospects for a cure have never been better.

James Lawrence, ninth grade. Spring musical. Bicycle club. Tennis club. School newspaper. Madrigals. Honor Society.

It's not his real name, but, yes, James Lawrence is a real kid—tall, arms and legs as long and skinny as a maple sapling, topped off with a handsome Hollywood "Brat Pack" face. And the only thing about him that smacks of underachievement is something he can't improve through study or sweat: his pancreas.

James has Type I, or insulin-dependent, diabetes. His pancreas—a solid, gourd-shaped gland wedged behind and slightly below his stomach—stopped making insulin when he was in the fourth grade. Because his body makes none of its own insulin, he must inject it into his skin twice every day.

Insulin is crucial to the body's use of food energy in the form of glucose, a blood sugar. Without glucose, the body's billions of cells would die of starvation.

Up until this century, a diagnosis of Type I diabetes meant a death sentence for every child who acquired the disease. Today, thanks to medical advances, nearly a million Americans—about half of them children and young adults, or 1 out of every 600 under age 20—are living with their diabetes. For most, that's quite an achievement. A child with diabetes is expected to learn and understand the subtle peaks and valleys of his or her own blood chemistry and to self-inject insulin two and sometimes three times a day. In effect, the child becomes, at 9 or 12 or 15 years old, his or her own doctor.

If your child has diabetes, of course, you know it isn't easy. But the child diagnosed today enjoys several advantages over children diagnosed even five years ago. For example:

- You aren't alone, Mom and Dad. Diabetes support teams—doctors, nurses, diabetes educators, nutritionists, and social workers—are at your beck and call.
- Revised exchange lists make it easier for your kid to *eat* like a kid.
- Exercise, along with aggressive blood sugar control, is perhaps your child's best hope of preventing or delaying the frightening complications of diabetes.

Nerve damage, gangrene, blindness, high blood pressure, amputations, stroke, heart and kidney disease—all are believed to be associated with the toxic effects of hyperglycemia, although the exact reasons are still unknown. But the diabetic child has something going for him: hope. The prospects for a cure have never seemed better. Although no one is making any promises, some leading scientists confidently predict that this generation may be the last to develop diabetes (see "Countdown to Cure" on page 259).

Why My Child?

It isn't too many sugary snacks that caused your child's diabetes, but a combination of two factors—heredity and an immune disorder. If parents are responsible, it is only through an unfortunate roll of the genetic dice.

Insulin-dependent diabetes, formerly known as juvenile diabetes, runs in families. Where this is the case, a child's chances of developing diabetes are higher. Boys are more likely to develop insulin-dependent diabetes than their sisters. Certain minority groups, blacks and native Americans, are less vulnerable than whites.

Only recently has Type I diabetes revealed itself to the probing eyes of scientists as an autoimmune disorder. It's a tragic case of mistaken identity. The body's immune de-

(continued on page 263)

Countdown to Cure

Is diabetes forever?

Maybe not. But, like the mythical grapes of Tantalus, a cure remains in sight but frustratingly out of reach. Still, some researchers boldly suggest that the end of diabetes may be near.

"The odds for a cure are excellent," predicts Noel Maclaren, Ph.D., a leading diabetes authority at the University of Florida at Gainesville. Dr. Maclaren believes a cure will be discovered before the turn of the century. "How much before that we're going to succeed, I'm not sure. My deadline is before my retirement—in 15 to 20 years."

Pioneering new treatments for diabetes are coming at a breathtaking pace. At this rate, such optimistic forecasts may bear fruit.

Until the definitive cure is found, and researchers find a way to prevent diabetes altogether, a number of new developments may offer hope to Type I diabetics and their families.

Here's a rundown of the latest technologies for the treatment of diabetes and its complications.

Pancreas Transplants

"I don't want to say what is a cure and what is not a cure," says David Sutherland, M.D., Ph.D., a surgeon at the University of Minnesota Hospital.

What Dr. Sutherland will say about the more than 170 pancreas transplants he has performed is that, in a number of cases, "they're off insulin, so they're no longer diabetic."

In this new procedure, a portion of a donor pancreas is implanted into the abdomen of the child with diabetes. The result, in many but by no means all cases, is a piece of healthy, insulin-producing pancreas in the transplant recipient.

(continued)

Countdown to Cure—Continued

That's the up side. Now the down side. In order to reduce the risk that the body might reject the transplanted pancreas segment, the patient must take immunity-suppressing drugs, such as cyclosporine and prednisone, for the rest of his or her life. This leaves the patient open to opportunistic germs and a slightly increased risk of cancer. Further, Dr. Sutherland concedes, immunity-suppressing drugs may cause long-term harm, such as kidney damage.

The same risk applies to transplants of beta cells, which Dr. Sutherland and others—notably, Paul Lacy, M.D., of Washington University in St. Louis—have attempted with some success. The need for immunity-suppressing drugs is somewhat reduced for beta cell transplants, though not altogether. Nevertheless, Dr. Sutherland has hope.

Such transplants normally are not performed on children, mainly because very young patients have not yet developed complications such as nerve damage or kidney dysfunction. Complications generally take 15 to 20 years to develop. The transplants normally are done on patients who are just beginning to show signs of further problems. The average age of a transplant recipient, Dr. Sutherland says, is 30.

Aminoguanidine

Diabetic cells appear to age faster and become brittle because of a peculiar phenomenon known as cross-linking. In diabetics, molecules of glucose link up with protein to form an overall less-flexible animal. This causes blood vessel walls to clog and become hard, leading to atherosclerosis.

But Michael A. Brownlee, M.D., assistant professor of medicine and biochemistry at New York's Rockefeller University, has narrowed down a chemical compound called aminoguanidine. And what aminoguanidine seems to do is act as a linebacker,

blocking the encroachment of glucose into what is basically protein territory.

Dr. Brownlee and his colleagues have tested aminoguanidine on rats and found that it successfully prevented glucose/protein cross-linking. The substance is not available yet for humans.

Relaxation

Mind over glucose? Using relaxation techniques, researchers at Cornell University Medical College and Rockefeller University have taught five Type I diabetic patients to bring their blood sugar under better control.

Using biofeedback-assisted relaxation techniques over a four-month training period, the diabetic study participants reduced their stress levels and reduced the range of their otherwise up-and-down blood sugar.

Insulin Pump

Not widely used, the insulin pump can help some highly motivated people with diabetes maintain glucose levels closer to those of nondiabetic people. Insulin is injected into the skin through a catheter from a pump worn like a Walkman. But the patient has to maintain constant watch over blood sugar levels. It's also expensive—about $150 a month.

Oral Insulin

It's still in the research stage, but Medical College of Ohio researchers believe it's possible to encase insulin in plastic. This would enable diabetics to swallow the vital hormone instead of injecting it.

Normally, insulin can't be taken orally because digestive enzymes destroy it before it reaches the large intestine, where it can be absorbed. But biochemist Murray Saffran, Ph.D., Douglas Neckers, Ph.D., and

(continued)

Countdown to Cure—Continued

colleagues think they've solved that problem. "All we do is coat the medication with a plastic," says Dr. Saffran. The plastic shields the insulin from digestive enzymes in the small intestine. But once it gets into the large intestine, Dr. Saffran says, "the bacteria essentially punch holes into the plastic. Whatever is inside leaks out."

The plastic coating has been tested on rats, but not yet on humans. No one knows how well it will work in people, but preliminary results in rats suggest that oral insulin isn't as efficiently absorbed as injected insulin.

In the long run, though, the convenience of a pill may win out over the needle.

Diabetes Detection

Finally, what about children who don't have diabetes? Is there any way to determine whether your child might be diabetes-prone? Can the disorder be prevented?

Scientists are taking preliminary stabs at a diabetes detection test. At the University of Florida at Gainesville, Dr. Maclaren and colleagues have screened more than 5,000 schoolchildren in Florida's Pasco County for islet cell antibodies—named after the Islets of Langerhans, dwelling place of the insulin-producing beta cells.

Of the 5,000, 21 tested positive for one of the two known antibodies, and one developed diabetes before the year was out. Four others had low insulin levels and were expected to develop the disorder.

But the test isn't foolproof, and it's still too complicated for use by your local hospital's laboratory. "It's only being done in a few laboratories in the world," says Dr. Maclaren. "We are very hopeful it's going to be a useful marker for diabetes in children, but we still have a lot to learn."

If a child tests positive, what then? Can the onslaught of the antibodies be turned back?

Possibly, with immunity-suppressing drugs. But there are serious concerns about the harsh effects of such drugs in children. "Some of the drugs, like cyclosporine, are so toxic that one can't continue autoimmune treatment indefinitely," says Peter Chase, M.D., a University of Colorado physician also engaged in islet cell testing.

Nevertheless, since the life expectancy of a diabetic child is about 45, and he or she is likely to be burdened in later years by devastating complications, the possible benefits of autoimmune treatment may outweigh the potential harm.

fenses—normally unleashed against invaders like germs and viruses—instead launch seek-and-destroy missions against the body's own healthy insulin-producing beta cells. These beta cells are clustered, like bursts of buckshot, in regions of the pancreas called the Islets of Langerhans.

Picture these renegade antibodies as hunter-killer satellites. Their damage is allowed to occur through genetic markers called HLA-DR3 and HLA-DR4. People who have these genetic markers are predisposed to develop beta cell antibodies.

The war between the antibodies and the beta cells is a hopelessly lopsided war of attrition. As the betas begin to die off one by one, the pancreas produces less insulin (see "Signs and Symptoms" on page 264). Often, a virus, such as the otherwise innocuous flu bug, appears to weaken the beta cell defenses to the breaking point, leaving the remaining beta cells vulnerable to the invading antibodies.

With little or no insulin in the bloodstream, glucose—all dressed up with nowhere to go—rises to abnormally high levels in the blood and, from there, spills over into the child's urine. Like a magnet, the glucose attracts important minerals, which drain from the body rapidly through fre-

quent urination. This loss of minerals, coupled with cellular starvation, may make your child feel like he or she has the flu.

What Parents Can Do

Because James had begun feeling run-down and was going to the bathroom more often, his mother, Jean, thought he

Signs and Symptoms

For everything, there is a season. Apparently, so, too, for Type I diabetes. Most new cases of Type I diabetes develop between November and March. Researchers think this seasonal link may have to do with collapse of the body's insulin-producing systems triggered by a cold or the flu. In fact, the early symptoms of Type I diabetes may mimic the flu. They include:

- Rapid weight loss.
- Frequent urination.
- Extreme hunger.
- Increased thirst.
- Fatigue.
- Irritability
- Nausea and vomiting.

If your child develops these symptoms, call your pediatrician or family practitioner.

For more information, contact:

- American Diabetes Association, National Service Center, 1660 Duke Street, P.O. Box 25757, Alexandria, VA 22313; 1-800-ADA-DISC.
- Juvenile Diabetes Foundation, 60 Madison Avenue, New York, NY 10010-1550; (212) 889-7575.
- National Diabetes Information Clearinghouse, Box NDIC, Bethesda, MD 20892.

might have a bladder infection. She couldn't have known, but James's beta cells had already lost the war.

"I sort of pieced things together," says Jean, a psychologist.

Still thinking James's problem might be a bladder infection, she took him to see a pediatrician in their North Jersey community.

"He had been growing, so he was thinning out, but I hadn't noticed any major change in weight," she says. "When we got there, they put him on the scale before they did anything else. He had lost 9 pounds over one or two months. My heart sank. I didn't know what it meant. So then they did a urine test. Based on the urine test, they knew immediately. It was diabetes."

Glucose trickles into the urine at a point doctors call the "renal threshold"—when blood sugar levels creep up to 160 to 180 milligrams of sugar per deciliter of blood. A normal blood sugar reading ranges from 70 to 120 before eating and, because of the higher levels of glucose introduced by food, from 100 to 140 after meals.

James reacted to the diagnosis as any child of 9 might. "The first thing that came to me when they told me was something I had read in a book, that people with diabetes can't do things other kids can do, that it was like being paralyzed, physically handicapped," James recalls. "I thought diabetic kids had to sit out gym. Things like that. So I was really upset, scared, and confused."

James's mother and his father, Bill, a real estate executive, say they, too, went through a period of sadness and confusion.

"It took us a couple of years to learn how to manage. None of us knew anything about diabetes, so it took us a while to understand what the routine ought to be," Bill says. "There was a certain amount of frustration at first, learning to manage James's blood sugar, adjusting insulin doses, and so on. But within a year James was able to figure out the relationship between what he was eating and how much insulin to inject, what his blood sugar levels were."

How James and his family coped with diabetes demonstrates two things: One, diabetes is more than just a medical problem. It's a social monkey wrench jammed into the

works of an otherwise smooth-running family machine. Two, with aggressive medical and social therapy, a child with diabetes can thrive and his or her family can survive.

The Team Approach

After James's diagnosis, he was referred to Arthur Krosnick, M.D., medical director of the Princeton Diabetes Treatment and Education Center in Princeton, New Jersey. Dr. Krosnick, along with teaching nurses on his staff, taught James and his family what they needed to know to keep the diabetes under control. They also paid attention to the nonmedical aspects of James's diabetes.

The parents' long-term goal is to get their child to accept responsibility for his self-care. In a child three or four years old, this may not be possible. Parents will have to test the child's blood sugar, adjust insulin doses, and inject the insulin. But as the child grows older, diabetes educators like to see him or her taking over—with adult supervision, of course.

The first step toward self-sufficiency, for many children, is testing blood sugar.

"The child will often do the first blood glucose test and perhaps the insulin shot, here in my office," says Dr. Krosnick, also editor-in-chief of *Diabetes Forecast*, a publication of the American Diabetes Association. "There's no question that, by age 12 or older, they should take over from the very beginning. But I've seen 9-year-olds just as capable."

If your child resists, Dr. Krosnick advises, "Don't be the autocrat and say, 'Do this because I tell you to do it.' " Instead, try contracting. That is, work out a compromise with your child and work your way steadily toward full compliance.

"I really like most children to test blood glucose four times a day," says Dr. Krosnick, "but most children are only willing to test about eight times a week. We ask the child if he or she would be willing to test two times a day. If the answer is yes, then I say, okay, we have a contract."

There are two important benefits. "One," says Dr. Krosnick, "we have a better idea of what the kid's glucose

is doing, and, two, we get the kid to take responsibility for his or her own care."

At the same time, Dr. Krosnick says, it's also important that the family understand that the child's diabetes is not just a health problem but an emotional burden on the whole family.

"We've found that children with diabetes often have an abnormal self-image. They feel they are damaged. Even if it doesn't come out externally, it can be a latent problem."

It's important to reassure the child that life can and will go on. "We continue to stress to diabetic children that they can indeed be normal in most aspects of living," says Dr. Krosnick. "We explain to them why they don't feel well. And we explain that as long as they keep this blood chemistry under control, they can do all the things they did before."

Not surprisingly, children and families who enjoy the aid and comfort of friends, relatives, and diabetes educators tend to cope quite well. That's one reason why the American Diabetes Association stresses a team approach to diabetes management.

Jean Betschart, a diabetes nurse-educator at the Children's Hospital of Pittsburgh, is herself a Type I diabetic. She's lived with the disorder for 20 years, since she was 18 years old.

"A lot of times we see parents from outlying areas, small towns, patients of pediatricians or family practitioners who haven't had the resources available to them at a medical center," says Betschart. "And those people often are very surprised to find out what really is available."

What's available, in numerous areas of the country, are diabetes care teams, with nurse-educators available to answer phone calls about insulin mixing and diet, or just to allay fears. They also teach diabetic children to do what they have to do—check blood sugar, mix insulin, take injections—and update them when they develop problems. "We're pretty much in constant touch," says Betschart.

"The people who have a diabetes care team available to them and who are able to utilize these supports tend to do better," says Betschart, who with fellow nurse-educator

Linda Siminerio has written an easy-to-understand guide for parents called "Children with Diabetes." It's available from the American Diabetes Association.

For those who don't have access to such a team, the support of family and friends can be just as important. Parents who go it alone often cope badly.

According to Betschart, who with Siminerio conducted a study of 150 such parents, the negative reactions include "crying, screaming, getting angry at your spouse, running out of the house, swearing, drinking, smoking, and yelling at the kids."

Parents and families who communicate with each other, who confide their fears and doubts, who work with the diabetes care teams or turn to God for comfort, seem to have a more solid, positive outlook.

One final word to fathers: You're a part of the team, too. "Often the father plays no role at all," says Dr. Krosnick, "and the burden is all on the mother. Right from the beginning we say, it's not the child's problem, it's the family's problem."

Nutrition for Diabetic Kids

The nutritional focus for diabetics has changed. Once it was thought that nothing was worse for diabetics than sugar. Now it's realized that sugar may not raise blood sugar any more than many other foods the diabetic normally eats.

Ice cream for the diabetic? Fast food? Once strictly on the Not Wanted list, these foods now are accepted, but only in small portions as occasional snacks.

Once proteins were considered to be the most important food group on the diabetic meal plan. Now proteins take a back seat to starches. What's happened?

In 1986, the American Diabetes Association, in cooperation with the American Dietetic Association, revised the 1979 nutritional recommendations to take into account the latest research. Here's what the parent has to know.

Growth. Your diabetic child is not on a diet. Rather, there should be a meal plan designed to encourage normal growth. "Our first recommendation for children, above any other, is that they eat a diet of sufficient calories and

nutritional content to maintain normal development," says Aaron I. Vinik, M.D., chairman of the Diabetes Association's Committee on Food and Nutrition and a contributor to the new recommendations. "Restricting a child's calories is totally unacceptable."

Carbohydrates. These are starches and sugars, like breads, beans, corn, cereals, pasta, crackers, and snacks like popcorn or pretzels. Also included, occasionally, are refined sugar, either alone or in such foods as ice cream, cookies, granola bars, or cake.

Carbohydrate intake should amount to 55 to 60 percent of total calories. "We changed the emphasis here," says Dr. Vinik. "In the past, the meat and protein exchanges were most important, but not any more. The reason is that most of the meats Americans eat are high in fat. We are recommending a reduction of fat intake to less than 30 percent of the caloric intake."

How about fiber? Although high-fiber foods are recommended for adults, there's no such endorsement for children. "We don't yet know the impact of high fiber on growing children," Dr. Vinik explains.

Protein. Emphasize poultry, fish, and lean to medium-fat red meats. Bake or broil—don't fry. Don't bread or coat meats. Use cooking spray, not butter or margarine, to coat pans.

Timing. It's crucial that your diabetic child eat regularly to help prevent precipitous peaks or valleys in blood sugar levels. Plan three daily meals, one or two between-meal snacks, and one bedtime snack.

Before you put your child on any meal plan, check with your doctor. It's also recommended that you meet with a nutritionist every three to six months to reevaluate the diet.

Working Out

Like many average American kids who spend too much time in front of the tube and not enough time working up a sweat, your child may resist the motion notion. Exercise is important for all of us, but there is increasing evidence that working out pays off for children with diabetes, and for a number of reasons.

A happy, healthy heart. Regular exercise strengthens

all muscles, including the heart. It reduces heart attack risks and lowers cholesterol (*Pediatrics*).

Insulin sensitivity. Well, maybe. Some reports do suggest insulin requirements are lower for diabetic kids who exercise (*Diabetes Therapy*).

But others aren't so sure. Says Dr. Vinik, "Studies have shown that exercise and calorie restriction do help overweight people lower glucose and sensitize their bodies to insulin. But the diabetic who is lean or of normal weight will have to adjust his or her insulin intake."

Until the question is resolved, regular exercise does have other measurable benefits. Regular physical activity may ultimately prove to increase insulin sensitivity for everyone.

Fewer complications. Diabetics who exercise appear to have significantly fewer strokes and amputations. Their blood pressure seems to be somewhat better than that of those who don't exercise.

Most important, diabetics who exercise are three times less likely to die after 25 years with the disease than diabetics who are not active (*Pediatrics*).

Enthusiasm. It's hard to measure scientifically, but a kid who is disciplined enough to exercise may be more conscientious about all the other aspects of diabetes self-care. "People who exercise feel better about what they're doing and how they adhere to complicated regimens," says Dr. Vinik.

For all of the above reasons, regular exercise is an important component of diabetes care for your child. But, as always, there are cautions.

Your doctor should know about and approve your child's exercise routine. For one thing, says Dr. Vinik, exercise may cause hypoglycemia, or low blood sugar. Food intake and insulin doses may have to be adjusted. If exercise has your doctor's okay, let the games begin.

Hope Springs Eternal

As researchers chip away at the enigma that is Type I diabetes, children with the disease and their families wait—and hope. But how much hope is healthy?

There is always the danger that the hope will not be realized before severe complications set in. What if a cure is found, but it's too late to help? What if a means is found to prevent diabetes in kids who don't yet have it, but no treatment is developed for those who have lived with diabetes for years?

"When I first got diabetes, they said there would be a cure in ten years or less," says James Lawrence. "Five years later, they're still saying ten years. In my opinion, that's not a good thing to tell a kid with diabetes. You've gotta have some hope, but they keep adding on."

As a parent, your principal concern—after a healthy kid—is a happy kid. On that score, most diabetic kids seem content, according to a long-term study of Pittsburgh area diabetic children conducted since 1978 by Maria Kovacs, Ph.D., associate professor of psychiatry at the University of Pittsburgh.

"There is no such thing as a diabetic personality. We've pretty much proven that notion to be false," says Terri Schnell, who has worked on the study with Dr. Kovacs. "Basically, these kids are surprisingly adaptive [to diabetes], probably more than people give them credit for being."

But what do you say when your child asks, "How much longer, Dad?" "A lot of parents do promise a cure," says Schnell. "But my gut reaction is that parents should not make promises they can't keep. Children have a different perception of time. When you say 'near future,' they're looking at next week. It's more important to stress to the child that although diabetes is a serious illness, it's a controllable illness. Parents should stress that compliance with nutritional and medical advice is probably the best guarantee for a healthy future."

Jean Betschart agrees. "That's what I tell the kids," she says. "You don't want to be falling apart when they come up with a cure. But I never make guarantees."

So the key here is, give children enough hope so they remain positive and optimistic. And the same advice applies to parents. No one can blame you for hoping for a cure.

Says James's mother, Jean, "Whenever there's a chance

to make a wish, blowing out birthday candles or whatever, that's what the wish is."

Recommended Reading

Here are some books worth reading.

Children with Diabetes, by Linda M. Siminerio and Jean Betschart (published by the American Diabetes Association, Alexandria, Virginia).

Diabetes: A New and Complete Guide to Healthier Living for Parents, Children and Young Adults Who Have Insulin-Dependent Diabetes, by Lee Ducat and Sherry Suib Cohen (published by Harper & Row, New York).

Kids, Food and Diabetes, by Gloria Loring (published by Contemporary Books, Chicago).

PART X: THE BIG PICTURE IN 1989

CHAPTER 37

100-Plus Tips for Tip-Top Health

Fresh advice on everything from arthritis to healthy sex, from America's leading health centers.

To keep on top of health advice, you've got to go to the top—to the treatment specialists. That's what we've done here. First, we combed the country for outstanding specialty clinics and hospital centers. Then we contacted the directors and other key medical personnel. Our mission: to glean the best, most current advice on today's most common health concerns. So, now, if you've got the time, we've got the best tips modern medicine has to offer. (*Note:* These tips are intended to supplement, not replace, the advice of your personal physician. If you suffer from chronic pain, cancer, high blood pressure, heart disease, or any other serious condition, discuss these suggestions with a qualified specialist who understands your individual case.)

Pain Relief

Shealy Institute for Comprehensive Pain and Health Care, Springfield, Missouri, C. Norman Shealy, M.D., Director

Ask your doctor about tryptophan. This amino acid is currently one of our top ten aids for pain relief. It can be remarkably useful in treating migraine, backache, neuralgia, and dental pain. Tryptophan converts into the neurotransmitter serotonin, which regulates sleep, increases pain tolerance, and relieves depression partly by activating beta-endorphins, the brain's natural opiates. Although it's nearly free of side effects, you shouldn't supplement your intake without a doctor's approval and supervision.

Alternate heat and ice. Hot and cold compresses used alternately (15 minutes each) are highly effective pain relievers.

Get three independent opinions before undergoing back surgery for pain relief. Back surgery ranks high among the most unnecessary surgeries.

Ask your doctor about colchicine. This is an antigout drug that is effective for back pain—and is safe even for people with ruptured disks. It acts as an anti-inflammatory, boosting your levels of prostaglandin E1, one of the body's natural pain relievers.

Stop smoking! Smokers tend to have twice as much pain as nonsmokers, possibly since smoking stimulates adrenaline, which sensitizes you to pain. Nicotine also blocks one of your body's natural pain relievers.

Cut out caffeine. Like smoking, caffeine stimulates adrenaline, which sensitizes you to pain.

Ask your doctor about TENS. Eighty percent of acute pain sufferers and 50 percent of chronic sufferers are helped considerably by transcutaneous electrical nerve stimulation, or TENS. Small battery-powered machines worn externally deliver a mild electric current to nerves without piercing the skin.

Boston Pain Center, Spaulding Rehabilitation Hospital, Gerald M. Aronoff, M.D., Director

Don't just sit there: Exercise! A sedentary lifestyle leads to a vicious circle of weak muscles and more pain whenever you do exert yourself. So work out to build muscle strength. Remember: Some discomfort while exercising is to be expected. Sensible exercise will pay off in the long run with reduced pain.

Try an ice massage. Freeze water in an empty margarine tub, then rub the skin directly, using a circular motion, for 5 to 10 minutes. The relief lingers anywhere from 30 minutes to 4 hours. Cold numbs, prevents or reduces swelling and bleeding, and inhibits the release of histamines, which promote inflammation and pain. (*Note:* Don't massage with ice if you have Raynaud's disease, peripheral vascular disease, or hypersensitivity to cold. And be sure to ask your doctor or physical therapist before trying this remedy at home.)

Diamond Headache Clinic, Chicago, Seymour Diamond, M.D., Director

Try cold compresses. If the headache doesn't go away, switch to heat. It's difficult to say whether a headache will respond to heat or to cold packs. In our experience, it has nothing to do with the nature of the pain. Although you'd think tension headaches (mainly muscular in origin) would respond to heat and migraine (mainly vascular) headaches to cold, our experience shows it's really an individual matter.

Keep regular hours. If you tend to get headaches when you're on vacation, when you're jet-lagged, or when you oversleep on weekends, stick to a routine. Try to wake up at the same time every day. Erratic sleep patterns can cause headaches.

Don't skip meals. Going hungry lowers blood sugar levels and can bring on hunger headaches.

New England Center for Headache, Cos Cob, Connecticut, Randall Weeks, Ph.D., Director of Research and Training

If you rely heavily on over-the-counter painkillers for frequent headaches, see your doctor. Our studies found that while analgesics are helpful in low doses, habitual use may paradoxically perpetuate headache pain. Caffeine constricts the blood vessels, providing temporary relief, but habitual use could cause rebound dilation and withdrawal headaches.

Lehrman Back Center, Miami, Florida, David Lehrman, M.D., Founder and Director

Make love! Back pain is exacerbated by tension, and many people tend to withdraw when they're in pain, which only makes things worse. Sex is a wonderful antidote. Not only is pelvic thrusting an ideal exercise for back strengthening, but orgasmic release is an excellent tension reducer.

Lighten up; don't be so serious. Laughter eases tension, promotes breathing, circulation, and muscle tone, and may even release chemicals that diminish pain. It also helps my patients stick to their program!

Weekend athletes: Ease up on your ego! If you are highly competitive, you're much more likely to sustain an injury or exacerbate your back problem. So play sports for fun, and don't knock yourself out when you start feeling physically or mentally fatigued.

Learn back-safe ways to play your sport. It's simply foolhardy to remain sedentary all week yet expect to golf, jog, or play tennis without pain on the weekend. Learn how to stay in shape, use proper form and good alignment, and warm up and cool down to protect your back.

Shower before you exercise! Hot water warms up your muscles enough to loosen them for exercise.

Sitting too long? Try this. Lie on the floor on your back with your knees well bent. Place a thin pillow under your neck and head and prop up your legs across the seat of a chair. Many people find that if they can get into this posture immediately for 5 or 10 minutes when they feel a backache coming on, they can circumvent or at least minimize the pain.

Boosting Immunity

Immunogenetics and Immunochemistry Laboratories, Washington, D.C., Terry M. Phillips, Ph.D., D.Sc., Director

Avoid irritations. Suppressing the immune system is easy to do—especially inadvertently. Constant physical irritations—such as a poorly fitted cast or occupational exposures to toxic chemicals—can slow your immune functions.

Keep a journal. Writing about painful personal problems and how you feel about them not only reduces stress

but may bolster the immune system, too. A study of college students showed that daily diary keepers who wrote about such things increased their infection-fighting white-blood-cell responses significantly over those who recorded thoughts on trivial subjects. The improved immunity held up six weeks later.

Don't skimp on sleep. Sleep is the repair shop for the body's immune system. During sleep, the immune system can use the energy reserves left over from the body's needs during the day. Without enough sleep to revitalize you, you become more vulnerable to infection.

Breathe through your nose, not your mouth. Nasal hairs can effectively filter out some of the 20 billion particles of foreign matter the average person inhales daily.

Quit smoking. Smoke paralyzes the tiny cilia (hairs) in the respiratory passages so that they become too limp to filter airborne germs.

When pressure builds, take a walk. Competition can become an immune-system stressor if you let it get to you. Studies show that medical students' immune functions become depressed during exam periods and take about three weeks to recover to normal. When too much pressure builds up, take a walk—or indulge in any other diversion that you find pleasurable enough to relieve the tension.

Find a quiet place to work—or use earplugs. Noise is a real immunity stressor. Your immune system requires a good measure of peace and quiet to recoup its resources.

Healthy Sex

Masters and Johnson Institute, St. Louis, Missouri, William H. Masters, M.D., Consultant

Check the drugs you take. Prescription drugs are a common cause of impotence and lack of sexual desire, especially in older men. The most common offenders are blood pressure drugs, including diuretics and vasodilators.

Don't try to be "normal." "Normal" is what works for you.

Get help if you're anorgasmic. Most women who are unable to have an orgasm during sexual intercourse can

learn to do so. Therapy varies according to each case, with success rates at 80 to 85 percent.

Talk—and make sure you listen. Most "sex" problems are really problems of intimacy and communication. Sharing uncertainties, worries, and other personal problems with a partner is essential for the growth of intimacy. Learn what it feels like to be talking in a trusting and honest way. Get help from a therapist if necessary.

Marriage Council of Philadelphia, Martin Goldberg, M.D., Director

Don't mix alcohol with sex. Alcohol may ease inhibitions, but it kills performance.

Weight Control

New England Deaconess Hospital's Nutritional Coordinating Center, Division of Eating Disorders, Boston, George L. Blackburn, M.D., Ph.D., Director of Nutrition Support Services

Find the fat in your diet and eliminate it. The body is genetically imprinted to accept fats and carbohydrates according to a set ratio. If you limit your diet to just 10 to 20 percent fat, your body automatically limits the amount of carbohydrate calories you can comfortably consume. This makes it impossible to gain weight. You can get fat only by eating too much fat.

Go the distance. Thirty minutes of aerobics three times a week is fine for cardiovascular fitness. But for weight loss, duration and frequency are more important than intensity. You're better off working out less strenuously five to seven days a week. Aim for 40 minutes of walking a day.

Avoid too-fast food. The faster you eat, the greater the tendency to overeat. It takes 20 minutes for the brain to get the message that the body's been fed and signal the appetite sensors that you've had your fill. If you down your meal in 5 minutes, you'll never get the feedback you need to know when to quit—until after it's too late.

Pregnant and overweight? Don't give in to your cravings till the last half of the pregnancy. Energy expenditure doesn't really increase until the last 12 weeks.

Weight gained in the first trimester is fat; it's tough to shed later, after the baby is born.

The Eating and Weight Disorders Clinic, Johns Hopkins Hospital Medical Institutions, Baltimore, Maryland, Arnold E. Andersen, M.D., Director

Think of your diet like you do your electric bill. If instead of paying $80 a month, you could write a check for $72, would you bother? Sure you would. When you annualize, the savings can be enormous. Likewise, a 10 percent cut in fat can add up to significant calorie savings over the course of a year.

Consider meat a luxury item. Most cuts of meat deliver a high percentage of their calories in the form of fat. To reduce your intake, do what people do where meat is a luxury item: Use it in moderation, to accompany a main course of vegetables, grains, or pasta.

Eat one-quarter to one-third of your daily calories at breakfast. If you skip breakfast, you may not hear rumblings until late in the day, but then hunger comes like an express train. If you find it difficult to stuff your face first thing in the morning, take a midmorning breakfast break. It will help curb that midafternoon overindulgence.

Fair Oaks Hospital Eating Disorder Program, Summit, New Jersey, Jeffrey Jonas, M.D., Medical Director

Change your behavior before your attitude. You can eventually lose cravings for certain foods, but not until bad habits have been broken. Besides, if you wait around until you really feel ready to sacrifice that nightly bowl of ice cream, you may never do it.

University of California Medical Center, Orange, California, Grant Gwinup, M.D., Chief of Endocrinology and Metabolism.

Swimming is good for your heart—but don't depend on it for weight loss. Swimming provides an excellent cardiovascular workout, but it doesn't compare to walking or cycling for weight loss. My study found that six months of daily workouts (of 1 hour each) led to a 10 percent weight loss for walkers, 12 percent for cyclists, and a slight weight gain for swimmers, even though they maintained a

stable diet. So if you have to lose weight, use some other form of exercise instead of or in addition to swimming.

Sharp Senses

Laboratory for Nutrition and Cataract Research, Tufts University, USDA Human Nutrition Research Center on Aging, Boston, Allen Taylor, Ph.D., Director

Take C and see. In animal studies, dietary vitamin C seems to concentrate in the lens of the eye, and may help protect it from sun damage. Vitamin C has also helped to prevent cataracts. Vitamin E may offer similar protection.

University of Houston, College of Optometry, Houston, William R. Baldwin, O.D., Ph.D., Dean

Go incognito. Sunglasses that protect your eyes from the sun's harmful ultraviolet light can help prevent cataracts. Look for glasses designated Z80.3. These glasses will filter out 95 percent of the harmful rays.

Get tested for glaucoma. After age 40, you should have your eyes examined for glaucoma every two years. Begin testing earlier if you have a family history of glaucoma or are black, diabetic, or taking cortisone or blood-pressure medication. Incidentally, while ocular pressure tests have been used routinely to diagnose glaucoma, visual field tests are now considered desirable for a full diagnosis.

Wills Eye Hospital, Philadelphia, William Tasman, M.D., Ophthalmologist-in-Chief

Blink, and blink again. You may notice it when you're reading or looking at a computer screen. You're so riveted to the image that you "forget" to blink. As a result, the surface of your eye dries out and becomes irritated. People with soft contact lenses, which require a lot of moisture, may also find that their vision blurs. So make it a point to blink regularly while you're doing concentrated work.

Peruse a landscape. Take a break from close-up work or reading to gaze out a window or across the room. Set your sights on some large, distant object—say, a rooftop swimming pool or the coffee cart. Give your eye muscles a stretch every hour or so to save them from fatigue.

Monell Chemical Senses Center, Philadelphia, Morley Kare, Ph.D., Director

Use it or lose it. Not everyone's ability to smell and taste declines with age. Professional perfumers usually get better with age and have the paychecks to prove it. Does their sense of smell remain sharp because it's been exercised over the years? It's possible, say the experts, that you can train your brain to be more attuned to input from your nose. And that's something it doesn't forget.

Eat around. The longer your senses are exposed to the same stimulus, the less "sensitive" they become. To avoid this sensory monotony, vary your diet. At meals, alternate food with every bite. And try a completely different taste between courses. A vinegary salad or light sorbet will release your taste and smell systems from boredom and perk them up for the next course.

University of Washington Medical School, Department of Otolaryngology, Seattle, Charles W. Cummings, M.D., Chairman

If you have to shout, get out. When you have to raise your voice just to carry on a conversation, the environment is noisy enough to damage your hearing in time.

Ears ringing? Switch pain relievers. Aspirin and related compounds can cause temporary, reversible hearing loss. It's nothing to worry about. But if it becomes bothersome, switch to a different kind of anti-inflammatory drug.

Don't put anything smaller than a baby elephant in your ears. Most ears are self-cleaning. The wax is pushed out by the new growth of ear-canal skin. If your ears aren't, use ear-cleaning drops or see your doctor.

Smell and Taste Center, University of Pennsylvania Hospital, Philadelphia, Richard Doty, Ph.D., Director

Butt out for good. Cigarettes can dull your senses of taste and smell. That's why people who quit are often amazed at how good food really tastes!

Use nasal sprays sparingly. Overuse of nasal sprays can produce dryness and other problems associated with smell loss. They may also permanently injure smell receptors. Don't abuse them. Follow manufacturer's directions.

Heart Health

Boston University Medical Center, Section of Preventive Medicine and Epidemiology, Joseph Stokes, M.D., Professor

Snack on fruit. Obesity is a prime risk factor for heart disease, and fruit will fill you up without filling you out. Eating fruit may also lessen your cravings for fatty foods, the real body-weight culprits (see the section on weight control).

Eat more oats and beans. The water-soluble fiber in these foods is effective in lowering cholesterol.

Order fish when you eat out. Make eating fish a habit at home, too. Have at least two fish meals a week to ensure an adequate supply of omega-3 fatty acids, which help lower your blood's cholesterol.

Make that saltwater fish. Saltwater fish, especially the dark-meat varieties, contain more beneficial oils. Freshwater fish with lighter meat contain relatively little oil.

Shellfish are good for your heart. Shrimp, lobster, and other crustaceans were once thought to be high in cholesterol. Actually, they're no worse than lean meat, and nowhere near as cholesterol-laden as liver and other organ meats.

Ask your doctor about aspirin. Some people may benefit from a daily dose. It's especially protective against strokes, and there is some evidence that aspirin may reduce the risk of a second heart attack in coronary patients.

Go Mexican (or Thai or Szechuan)! Onions, garlic, and hot peppers contain substances that thin your blood, lower your blood pressure, and reduce your cholesterol levels.

Boone Hospital Center, Columbia, Missouri, Tom La Fontaine, Ph.D., Director of Cardiac Rehabilitation

Use up 2,000 to 3,500 calories a week. That should include 30 to 45 minutes, three to five days a week, of aerobic activity at your target heart rate (determined by test results), plus a total of 1 hour a day of physical activity. You can count the minutes you climb stairs, walk, mow the lawn or garden—as long as they add up to an hour a day.

Warm up and cool down. Sudden starts and stops tax your heart and your muscles. For safety's sake, spend at

least 5 to 10 minutes before your workout getting your circulation going, and afterward gradually decrease your activity until your heart returns to close to its resting rate.

Ease up on the competition. Work out to have fun and get healthy, but don't push beyond burning 3,500 calories a week. Studies show the health benefits of exercise drop off after that point. Runners who do more than 30 miles a week start getting injuries and chronic fatigue. A number of coronaries have occurred among people who tried to outrow and outcycle their electronic targets on the new high-tech equipment.

Meyer Friedman Institute in Mount Zion Hospital and Medical Center, San Francisco, Meyer Friedman, M.D., Director

Analyze your stress style. Do you: Clench your fist during ordinary conversation? Play to win even in trivial contests with children? Get angry easily? Have trouble sitting and doing nothing? Detest waiting in lines? Eat, walk, or talk fast? Grind your teeth? If you habitually do at least one of these, it's time to take stock. These are considered type-A habits—cardiac risk factors that can do you in as sure as an elevated cholesterol level.

Have a change of heart. Make a concerted effort to reverse your type-A habits. Don't wear a watch. Get in the longest checkout line when you're at the supermarket. Smile at other people and laugh at yourself. Play to lose, at least some of the time. Stop trying to think or do more than one thing at a time. Walk, talk, and eat more slowly. Do nothing but listen to music for 15 minutes each day. Cheerfully say "Good morning" to each member of your family and to people you see at work.

Arthritis

The Arthritis Foundation, National Office, Atlanta, Floyd Pennington, Ph.D., Group Vice-President for Education

Use creative problem solving. To break the stress/pain/depression cycle, learn to see your problems as challenges rather than limitations. If you can't reach the cereal box on the top shelf, put it on the bottom shelf or install

lower shelves. Find new ways to get around your difficulties; don't let them overwhelm you.

Cut back on salt. Sodium may cause swelling that can stress your joints.

Keep active. Many arthritis sufferers think they shouldn't be active. This may not be true for many arthritics! Exercise keeps your joints healthy. Disuse will only cause more pain in the long run. Walk, bike, swim, get your heart rate up. Ask your doctor about the best exercise for you.

Lose excess weight. Obesity is now regarded as a serious risk factor for some forms of arthritis.

Rheumatology Division, Department of Internal Medicine, University of Texas Medical Branch, Galveston, Emilio Gonzalez, M.D., Assistant Professor

Take all arthritis medications with meals. This will prevent or reduce the stomach irritation and/or upset associated with many arthritis medications, including aspirin. If your prescription calls for taking the medication more than three times a day, ask your doctor about amending the schedule. Today's new anti-inflammatory drugs are available in a wide range of doses that make possible much simpler prescribing schedules.

Make your morning shower a hot one. The moist heat reduces joint stiffness.

Take a course in laborsaving and stress-saving techniques. Specially designed for people with arthritis, these courses are taught by certified physical therapists. They can show you how to protect your joints without sacrificing one bit of your ability to perform everyday tasks. For more information, contact the nearest chapter of the Arthritis Foundation.

Depression

Western Psychiatric Institute and Clinic, Pittsburgh, Cleon Cornes, M.D., Medical Director, Depression Prevention Program

Know how much stress is best for you. Stress is a key factor in depression, but some people function best with a lot of stimulation, others with very little. Find how much you need to feel in control of your life.

Take major life changes one at a time. Major life changes—even good ones, like getting married or starting an exciting new job—can precipitate depression, especially when you take on more than one at a time. Take control by dealing with each major change individually. If you're relocating for a job, try to postpone your first day at work until you feel settled in your new home.

Get out your grief with tradition. Suppressing grief can add to the pain of your sadness and loss. You can draw great benefits from engaging in family rituals and ceremonies. Whether it's sitting shiva or holding a wake, centuries of tradition and custom offer socially acceptable ways to fully express your mourning. If you don't have a traditional outlet, create your own rituals with friends, family, or community.

Don't suffer in silence. Many people let their feelings of hopelessness and helplessness snowball into full-scale depression in the belief that no one can help them. But nearly 80 percent of depression is treatable. So when you feel the blues coming on, pick up the telephone and make a call to your minister, a counselor, or a friend, or ask your doctor for a referral to a qualified specialist.

Don't let anger simmer. Long-term, intense conflicts with family or friends are major contributors to depression. But don't walk away from your differences. Do your best to learn how to resolve arguments constructively so that both parties feel like winners.

Share and care. Depression feeds on loneliness and isolation. Create a support system so you can reach out to others. Even keeping a pet can help. Giving to others—whether it's to humans or animals—is a great stress reducer and antidote to depression.

Cultivate an exercise habit. Many depressed people report that daily workouts like swimming or jogging help them feel better. If you get started on a regular program when you have energy, it will be easier to stick to when you're feeling down.

Body Conditioning

Exercise Physiology Laboratory, University of Louisville, Bruce Gladden, Ph.D., Director

Make like a turtle. The slow but steady approach to exercise will keep you in the running. People who let their newfound enthusiasm overwhelm their common sense are more likely to drop out due to burnout, boredom, or injuries. So begin slowly, maybe by walking 15 minutes a day three to five times a week. Increase gradually, by 5 minutes a week. Of course, consult your doctor if you're over 35 and haven't worked out in years.

Use your belly to save your back. A strong midsection is the best protection against a bad back. Unfortunately, most people try to strengthen their stomachs the wrong way and put strain on their back in the process. Instead of traditional sit-ups, do "curls." Bend your knees, put your hands loosely on your shoulders, and then, slowly, without jerking, contract your stomach muscles and curl your chest and shoulders up off the floor. Don't sit up completely. Then, slowly lower down.

Do a double-take on pain. Learn the difference between muscle soreness and pain from an injury. Muscle soreness eases with exercise. Pain from an injury usually gets worse with exercise. Keep in mind, too, that if you ache after every workout, you are either exercising too hard or too infrequently. Either way, you are setting yourself up for serious damage.

Find an activity that fits your body. You'll be more likely to stick with a workout that accommodates (not ignores) your body's little foibles. If you're overweight, try swimming or pool exercise classes; fat floats in the water, lifting weight off stressed joints. If stiff muscles or arthritis slow you down, take up yoga or join a stretching class. If you have stamina to spare but feel flabby, try a light weight-lifting program. Of course, for almost everyone, regardless of age, weight, or condition, walking is usually a better investment of your exercise time. An aerobic exercise of some type is best.

Kenneth Cooper Aerobics Research Center, Dallas, Kenneth Cooper, M.D., Director

Be nice to your knees. Let's face it: When your knees say, "No way," you're not going anywhere. To prevent problems, strengthen the leg muscles that absorb shock and stabilize this joint. Best bets: bicycling and proper use of weight lifting on fitness equipment designed to work both the front and back of your legs. If, despite these preventive measures, you hurt a knee, rest it for a few days. If the pain persists, see your doctor. Knee braces will help only certain injuries, such as tendon or muscle strains.

Trade in your sneakers for a good pair of fitness shoes. Lots of time and money have been poured into making sports equipment that's better than ever. Case in point: shoes. Yesterday's multipurpose sneaker has given way to specialized shoes for walking, running, tennis, aerobics, you name it. These shoes are engineered for comfort and performance and to ease stress on feet and joints. So, after you've chosen your sport, invest in a good shoe to go with it.

Use vanity to your advantage. There's nothing wrong with a little narcissism, if that's what it takes to get your heart pounding to an aerobic beat.

Be patient. Don't expect too much too fast. In exercise studies, researchers typically follow participants six to eight weeks before significant drops in heart rate, blood pressure, and weight are noted. So don't quit before you've given your program a chance to take effect. Remember, you didn't get out of shape overnight. One consolation: The *more* unfit you are, the quicker you'll see results.

Find your steady state. You'll know it when you get there. It's your body's "sweet spot"—where your heart rate is elevated but steady; where you are breathing hard enough to make talking a little difficult; where you feel comfortably stressed and can sustain the pace for at least 20 minutes.

Cancer Prevention

Roswell Park Memorial Institute, Buffalo, New York, Curtis Mettlin, Ph.D., Director of Cancer Control and Epidemiology

Follow the ten commandments of cancer prevention. Eat more cabbage-family vegetables (including cauli-

flower, broccoli, and brussels sprouts). Add more high-fiber foods to your diet. Choose foods high in vitamin A. Do the same for foods high in vitamin C. Control your weight. Trim the fat from your diet. Limit salt-cured, smoked, and nitrite-cured foods. Stop smoking. Go easy on alcohol. Avoid overexposure to the sun. Through these measures, 50 percent of all cancers might be prevented.

Exercise. Recent studies suggest that exercise may guard against certain kinds of cancer in both men and women.

Learn the early warning signs. If everyone practiced early detection, we might double the cancer cure rate. Ask your doctor to familiarize you with the early warning signs and appropriate screening methods.

Dana Farber Cancer Institute, Boston, W. Bradford Patterson, M.D., Director of Cancer Control

Request information before surgery. People who know what to expect tend to be more confident and relaxed, which can promote recovery and may reduce complications.

Memorial Sloan-Kettering Cancer Institute, New York City, Jeanne A. Petrek, M.D.

Fight fear with facts. Due to recent advances, the facts about the diagnosis and treatment of cancer may be more encouraging than you think. Today, many operations are less extensive than they were previously.

National Surgical Adjuvant Breast and Bowel Project, University of Pittsburgh School of Medicine, Bernard Fisher, M.D., Director

Ask questions, shop around for a surgeon, and get a second opinion before breast biopsy, not afterward. Based on the size of the lump, its location, and a few other parameters, your physician should be able to determine whether you qualify for lumpectomy, a breast-sparing procedure. If you qualify, the lumpectomy can be done at the time of biopsy. This can save you additional surgery later should the lump prove cancerous.

Healthy Digestion

Digestive Diseases Laboratory at Memorial Hospital, Houston, Robert E. Davis, M.D., Director

Don't run on empty. When you skip meals or allow too much time between meals, acid builds up in your stomach, setting you up for dyspepsia—that gnawing, queasy feeling—which, over time, can develop into ulcers in some people.

Don't pacify hunger pangs with coffee. Coffee—including decaffeinated—increases acid in the stomach. So, while that cup of coffee after a meal may stimulate digestion, it may upset your stomach—or worse, precipitate an ulcer—when it's the only thing going down.

Don't take aspirin for a hangover. Aspirin can dramatically increase the irritation of a stomach already irritated by alcohol.

Prone to heartburn? Avoid chocolate, spearmint, and peppermint—as well as alcohol and fatty foods. These foods can interfere with the normal function of the valve that prevents the stomach contents from backing up into the esophagus.

Ask your doctor about Pepto-Bismol for ulcer relief. Several researchers have had great success healing ulcers and preventing their return with Pepto-Bismol. This common over-the-counter medication contains bismuth, a heavy metal that not only aids healing but also has antibacterial properties. Recent studies suggest that bacteria may be a contributing cause of some ulcers.

Stop smoking. People who smoke tend to have problems in their gastrointestinal tract. Smoking decreases bicarbonate production, which buffers acid in the stomach.

Limit alcohol intake. Unlike coffee, which stimulates acid secretion, alcohol is itself an irritant to the stomach lining. Taken with or after a meal, the effect is negligible. But on an empty stomach, alcohol can irritate and set your stomach lining up for inflammation, or even ulcers.

Ageless Skin

Aging Skin Clinic, University of Pennsylvania, Philadelphia, Albert M. Kligman, M.D., Ph.D., Director

Give your nose a lift. Long-term sun exposure can damage the cartilage in the nose, causing the tip to droop. In fact, it's the sun, not age, that's solely responsible for this. Sun exposure also causes enlarged, clogged follicles on your nose.

Give yourself some extra lip service. Lips don't have the protection of melanin the rest of your body has. They should always be protected by a high-SPF sunscreen in stick form. And the waxy consistency gives the sunscreen more lasting power to hold up to lip licks.

Wear sunglasses that absorb UVA light. They help protect the thin skin of your eyelids and area around your eyes.

Lead a shady life. We've said it before and we'll say it again: All prematurely aged skin is preventable. Just steer clear of the sun's rays—and protect yourself with a good sunscreen when you can't. Use a product with as high a sun-protection factor (SPF) as you can buy. And be sure to cover all exposed skin, even on those areas, like the soles of your feet or underside of your chin, where you'd think the sun doesn't shine. The fact is, when you're outside, the sun doesn't hit you like a spotlight: It comes at you from all directions as if you were submerged in a tub of radiation.

High Blood Pressure

The Helmsley Cardiovascular Center, New York Hospital-Cornell Medical Center, New York City, Thomas G. Pickering, M.D., Professor of Medicine

Have your blood pressure taken again . . . and again. Blood pressure can sometimes shoot upward in response to pretest stress. At least in cases where the blood-pressure reading is mildly high, taking the test again and again at regular intervals over a period of several months may remove enough apprehension about the test itself to produce a near-normal reading.

Slim down. Losing weight is as important as restricting salt.

Give dietary changes a chance. Sometimes a dietary switch—to less salt, fat, and alcohol and more fish and foods containing magnesium, calcium, and potassium—is

all that's needed to lower your blood pressure. But you've got to make a commitment to it. Give these dietary changes at least a month before turning to medication for high blood pressure.

Adopt health habits with double dividends. Consider other cardiovascular risk factors along with high blood pressure and tackle two or more at a shot. Regular aerobic exercise, for example, will not only lower your blood pressure, it will also have a favorable effect on blood lipids.

Premenstrual Syndrome (PMS)

Portman Clinic, Madison, Wisconsin, Edward Portman, M.D., Director

Ask your doctor about natural progesterone therapy. More commonly prescribed synthetic progesterones (called progestogens) and birth-control pills can actually make PMS symptoms worse.

Give lifestyle changes a chance. Sometimes, mild PMS responds to simple lifestyle changes, such as getting more exercise, consuming less salt and caffeine, and eating more nutrient-rich foods. If you find you can't control your behavior, you may have PMS more severely than you want to admit, or you may have something else. Seek medical help.

Make sure it really is PMS. Thyroid problems, low blood sugar, even disorders like manic depression can mimic PMS symptoms. Chart your symptoms over a few months to see if they're strictly premenstrual. And see an internist or gynecologist for a qualified diagnosis.

The Division of Reproductive Medicine at North Charles Hospital, a Johns Hopkins Medical Institution, Baltimore, Maryland, Robert S. London, M.D., Director

If you take vitamin B_6, reduce your dosage. Several small studies suggest that vitamin B_6 may relieve PMS symptoms, particularly depression. But large doses of this vitamin have been linked with reversible nerve damage.

Ask your doctor about vitamin E. In a recent study, women who took 400 international units of vitamin E for three months had a reduction in physical symptoms like

breast tenderness, weight gain, and abdominal bloating. They also had a reduction in mood symptoms, such as depression and anxiety. And they were less tired and had fewer headaches.

Restful Sleep

Sleep Disorders Center, Scripps Clinic, La Jolla, California, Merrill M. Mitler, Ph.D., Director of Research

Exercise according to a sleep schedule. A good workout can set the stage for a good night's rest—if you time it right. Mornings or late afternoons are best. Exercising just before retiring can be so invigorating that it keeps you wide-eyed and sleepless. (Sex doesn't count here; sex at bedtime can actually enhance sleep.)

Create a sleep sanctuary. Reserve your bed and bedroom for sleep and sex *only*. Consider your sleeping quarters off-limits for reading, watching TV, talking on the phone, writing letters, or worrying about tomorrow. These activities can clutter your "sanctuary" with associations that sabotage sleep.

Regulate your shuteye. Your sleep/wake cycle, that inner clock that tells you when to snooze and when to wake up, goes haywire when your sleep routine is disturbed. So become a creature of habit: Retire and rise at the same time and get the same amount of sleep every night. Consistency is the watchword for siestas, too: If you can't nap every day at an appointed time, don't nap at all.

Eat to sleep like a baby. The basic rules are simple: Don't eat a big meal before bedtime, but don't go to bed feeling hungry. A light bedtime snack should keep hunger at bay. Also, avoid caffeine after 4:00 P.M. and alcohol after 7:00 P.M.

Stop Smoking

Freedom from Smoking Clinic, American Lung Association, Jacksonville, Florida, branch, Chris Deputy, Director of Smoking and Health Education

Tell yourself why. It's estimated that 90 percent of smokers want out. The real trick is finding which reasons

will motivate you best. Set aside some time to think about why you want to quit. Make a list and read it daily until you feel ready to make the commitment.

Drink lots of water and fruit juice. Drinking fluids will help flush toxins from your system, shortening the withdrawal period.

Practice the four D's. When you feel the urge to smoke, try one of these: Take a deep breath, do something different, drink water or fruit juice, or delay the urge to smoke.

"Smoke" a cinnamon stick. People who feel addicted to the process of hand to mouth may find a cigarette substitute helpful. A cinnamon stick has a hole through the center, so you can "inhale" and get a pleasant cinnamon taste.

Smoking Cessation Program, Metropolitan Hospital, New York City, Alan Lipschitz, M.D.

Quit cold. Tapering down is virtually impossible for most smokers. People who try fail because the last remaining cigarettes become grossly overvalued.

If you've tried and failed, try again. Even a smokeless month or year is a victory. If you fall off the wagon, buck up and jump back on again. Remember, most successful quitters have a history of failed attempts.

Healthy Feet

Foot and Ankle Institute, Pennsylvania College of Podiatric Medicine, Philadelphia, Clare Starrett, D.P.M.

For warmth, waterproof boots are more important than fleece-lined ones. You can always warm up cold feet with an extra layer of socks. But damp feet are virtually impossible to warm up.

Vinegar stops odor and discourages athlete's foot. If you've got chronic athlete's foot or a foot-odor problem, bathe your feet three to four times a week in warm water laced with ½ cup of vinegar. The acidity inhibits fungus and odor-causing bacteria. If the odor persists after two weeks, ask your doctor about prescription ointments.

Hara Podiatrist's Group, Covina, California, Ben Hara, D.P.M.

Walk, walk, walk. Regular exercise keeps feet healthy, and walking is, by far, the best form. It strengthens foot muscles and improves circulation without putting excess stress on bones. Good circulation to the feet helps prevent a whole host of problems, including severe night cramping and intermittent claudication.

Step on the gas. Many people mistakenly think that circling the ankle exercises feet best. In fact, pumping the foot on an imaginary gas pedal does more to keep inner mechanics running smoothly. This motion causes the calf muscle to send blood coursing through the foot's veins and arteries.

Don't smoke. One cigarette can impair circulation for up to 45 minutes by constricting small blood vessels. The narrow vessels in the feet are particularly vulnerable to the damaging effects.

Foot Clinics of New York, New York College of Podiatric Medicine, New York City, Simon Nzuzi, D.P.M., Podiatric Medical Director

Bone up on calcium. It's easy to forget that osteoporosis can affect the foot's small bones as much as the skeleton's large ones. Brittle foot bones are susceptible to multiple fractures, which can make walking difficult and painful, if not impossible. Protect your future mobility by upping your intake of low-fat dairy products, tofu, broccoli, and leafy greens like collards, kale, mustard, and turnip greens.

Try a tea soak. If your feet perspire a lot, you'll be prone to nail problems. Try soaking your feet in black tea twice a day for 5 to 10 minutes. Continue for several days, tapering off as your condition improves. The tannic acid in tea has a drying effect. And dry toes resist ingrown nails better than moist skin, which is soft and easily penetrated. Consult a podiatrist if the condition persists.

High Anxiety

Massachusetts Mental Health Center Phobia Clinic, Boston, Robert M. Goisman, M.D., Director

Don't deny your fears and anxieties; flow with them. Fighting nervous feelings only worsens their effect. For example, the more you try to stop your hands shaking, the more anxious you'll become. The more anxious you become, the more your hands shake. The worry becomes a self-fulfilling prophecy. Try instead to observe anxious feelings in a detached, less emotional way. This may help to put your fears in perspective and, at the same time, alleviate those telltale physical signs.

Afraid to act? Do it anyway. There's an old saying that if you fall off a horse, get right back on. Fears fester unless you learn how to confront and master them. Just try to do it slowly: If you attempt to tackle your fears too quickly, you could create even more anxiety.

Work it out. Exercise burns off excess adrenaline. So, when the going gets rough, go for a walk.

Imagine yourself coping. Do you dread some upcoming event? If so, close your eyes and imagine yourself in that situation. Play it through: Imagine yourself coping or even enjoying it. This desensitization process will help prepare you for the real thing.

Outpatient Anxiety Disorders Clinic, Unit on Anxiety and Affective Disorders, National Institute of Mental Health, Bethesda, Maryland, Murray Stein, M.D., Administrator

Don't worry about things you can't control. Too many people worry constantly about problems they can never solve. Learn to act on problems that are within your power to resolve, and to not waste time worrying about those that aren't. In so doing, you'll quickly discover that most "worries" simply are not worth worrying about.

Think "challenge," not "crisis." Stressful situations can paralyze or stimulate you. It's all in how you look at things. People who handle stress well are those who have learned to approach the problems in their life as opportunities for personal growth—not as obstacles.

Index